ULRIKA DAVIDSSON

GREEN KICKSTARTS!
Metabolism Boosters
for Detox and
Weight Loss

PHOTOS BY ULRIKA POUSETTE

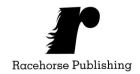

Racehorse Publishing

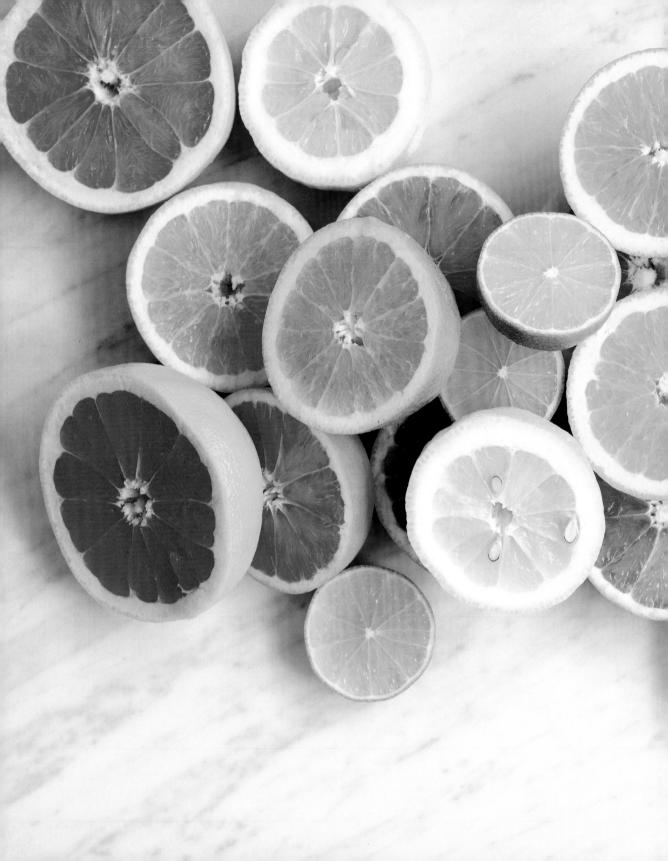

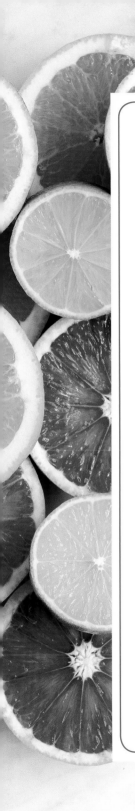

CONTENTS

FOREWORD

Kickstart Your Greener Life!

Welcome to the healthy world of vegetables. Here, I will provide you with inspiration for finding a vegetarian diet that fits you and makes you feel good.

Iceberg lettuce, corn, cucumbers, and tomatoes . . . vegetables are so much more than that. This book contains more than eighty recipes that are fresh, easy, and fun to prepare. Plus, they're free of gluten, cow's milk, and refined sugar.

There are lots of nutritious foods to enjoy: soups, salads, satisfying pie and gratin recipes, veggie burgers, raw food meals, and desserts free of refined sugar. This large variety of recipes offers many possibilities to find new favorites—now and in the future.

Many choose to go 100 percent vegetarian, but you can also be a "flexitarian" and eat vegetarian food once or a few times a week, which is how I eat. I happily eat vegetarian dishes but enjoy adding in a small amount of fish, shellfish, poultry, pork, lamb, and beef now and then.

There are many reasons to try a green kickstart, whether you're already a vegetarian or you've never cooked vegetarian. You'll get plenty of important vitamins, antioxidants, and essential fiber from vegetables and fruit. You also lower your body's pH level, which might lead to big improvements in health. Last but not least, a vegetarian diet helps protect our environment.

The kickstart menus in this book are perfect to follow over one to two weeks. You can then decide, after one or several completed kickstarts, how far you wish to take eating vegetarian meals.

I sincerely hope that you get plenty of green happiness from these recipes!

Ulrika Davidsson

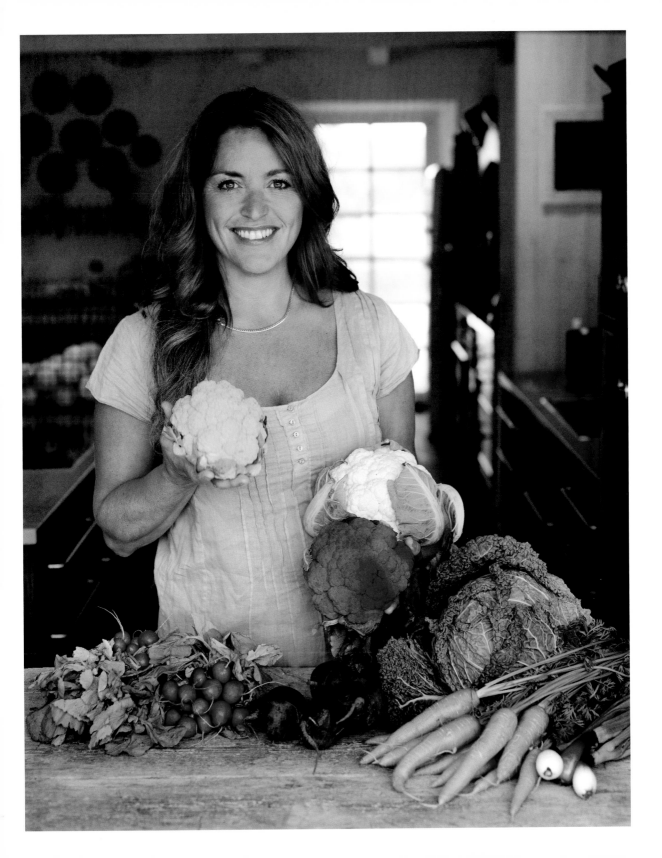

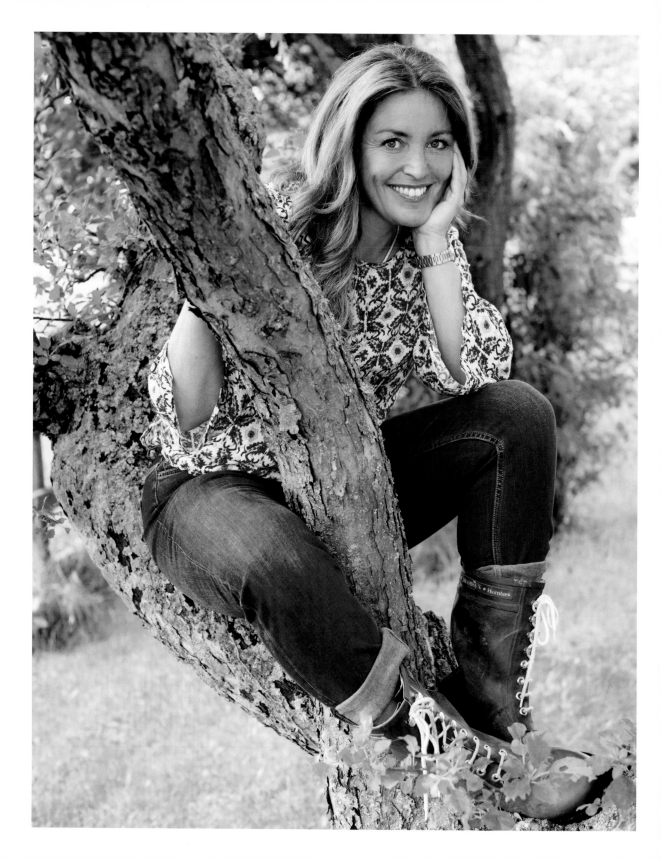

INTRODUCTION

What Is a Kickstart?

A kickstart is all about expending a little extra energy and effort getting started losing excess weight. You'll soon get your energy and strength back once you realize what a boost this is for your weight loss. The kickstart kicks right back! It will surprise you how much you can change your way of thinking, your needs, and the way you tackle challenges. And you'll discover new, delicious flavors, as well as needs and feelings that will help you in your long-term health changes.

While doing a kickstart you're going to concentrate on following the diet schedule to the letter and prepare yourself to skip all indulgences. It's far easier than you think, because the kickstarts in this book are long enough to show good results but short enough for you to follow them 100 percent successfully.

What's in a Kickstart?

Easy-to-prepare recipes that are filling, but more importantly, delicious. You'll get calorie-tabulated breakfasts, lunches, dinners, snacks, and desserts. The recipes are based on natural, raw ingredients and are almost all completely free of gluten and refined sugar. *A diet schedule* built from the chapters' recipes that provides you with all the information about when and what you should eat over one or two weeks. The menu is built on a low-carbohydrate food menu (see p. 10) combined with intermittent fasting (not applicable with juicing), and means that you'll be eating about 500 to 2,000 calories a day. The result could be weight loss of about 4½ to 11 pounds (2 to 5 kg).

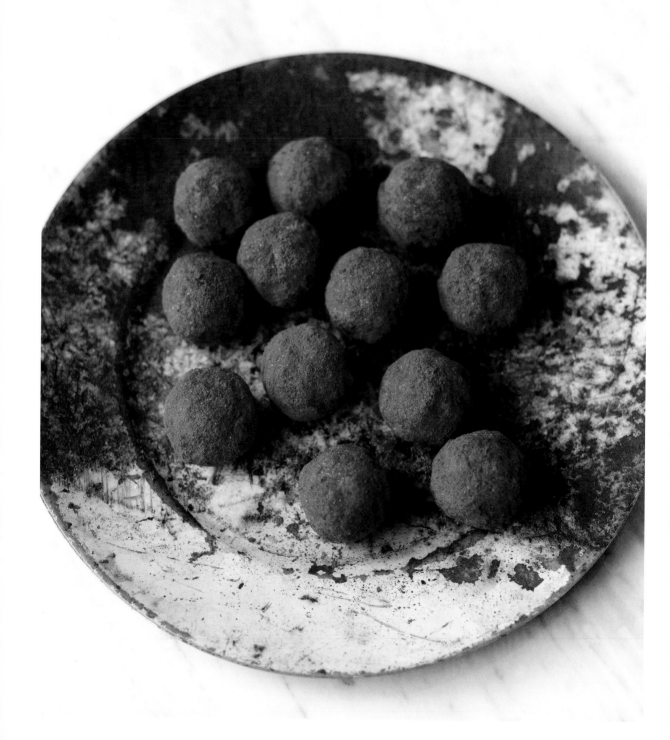

A KICKSTART GUIDE

Who are you and which kickstart is right for you? You yourself will know best because there is no diet or eating plan that suits everyone. We're all different, and we all have different needs. It makes a big difference whether you're young or old, if you're healthy or not, if you're sedentary or active, and if you're at a comfortable weight or if you're carrying excess pounds.

Read through the different diet schedules and take a look at the corresponding recipes. You'll soon see which of the four different kickstarts you prefer.

Detox is for those of you who aim to complete a two-week cleansing cure with vegetarian dishes free of gluten, dairy products, and refined sugar. The focus is on weight loss, but also on detoxing your body and providing the body's organs with relief in order to avoid gastrointestinal problems and bodily aches.

Vegetarian is for those of you who are curious about vegetarian dishes and want to learn how to combine a low-carbohydrate diet with intermittent fasting. The diet schedule lasts two weeks and provides the basics of vegetarian meal preparation, plus a kickstart for your weight, body measurements, and health!

Raw Vegan is suitable for those of you who want to try raw food meals and vegan dishes. Raw means that you don't heat food above 107.6°F (42°C). The vegan dishes are of course made without animal protein, but are also free of gluten, cow's milk, and eggs. This is a weeklong diet schedule that will provide good insight into this particular lifestyle and the recipes that will enable you to begin.

Juicing is for those of you who want to go through an effective weeklong body cleanse. Here the focus is on consuming smoothies, vegetable and fruit juices, and satisfying vegetable soups. This kickstart will give you a lighter body and lots of energy and is recommended for anyone who is curious about juicing and all its beneficial effects.

A Low-Carbohydrate Diet and Intermittent Fasting
—AN EFFECTIVE COMBINATION

All kickstart schedules in this book are based on the popular low-carbohydrate diet—or nutritional plan, as I prefer to call it. Many have successfully lost excess weight on this diet, and it's easy to understand why. Here I want to share experiences—my own and those of many others—to give you an understanding of why you will eat this way during your kickstart.

After working for a long time as a personal coach as well as a weight-loss group leader, I have clearly noticed that this type of lifestyle does work wonders for most people if they consume plenty of vegetables and the right amount of carbohydrates. It is, among other things, about you as a person, your lifestyle, how carbohydrates affect you, and if you prefer more or less fat in your diet. I myself eat a relatively low amount of carbohydrates, and use both saturated and unsaturated fats as long as they're natural.

The low-carbohydrate lifestyle works well for me and for so many others because it increases the body's fat metabolism while decreasing the fat cells' ability to store fat. So, how does this work? Well, all the carbohydrates we consume, whether in the form of sugar or starch, like in bread or pasta, for example, are broken down in the intestine and converted to glucose (dex-trose). Then the glucose travels via the blood into our cells to provide us with energy. Blood sugar rises to help push the glucose into the cells, while insulin is released to lower the blood sugar again. The more carbohydrates we eat, the more insulin is produced to lower the blood sugar level.

At the same time, insulin indicates that the body now has a lot of energy, that we are well nourished. The body then chooses to save body fat for a later time when it will be needed. High insulin levels also contribute to lower fat burning, since the body is using the glucose created by the carbohydrates we ate as fuel.

Carbohydrates are the quickest nutrient for the body to break down, and are the easiest to convert to glucose energy. Converting fat and protein to glucose energy is a far more complex process that requires more energy. If we consume lots of carbohydrates, instead of being slotted as energy into the cells, the excess glucose that is generated will be converted to fat that is stored in the fat cells. Excess glucose can also generate increased stress and raise the risk of inflammation in the body. Instead, with a low-carbohydrate diet the body starts to use stored fat. Quite simply, the body prepares itself to use a higher amount of fat for energy.

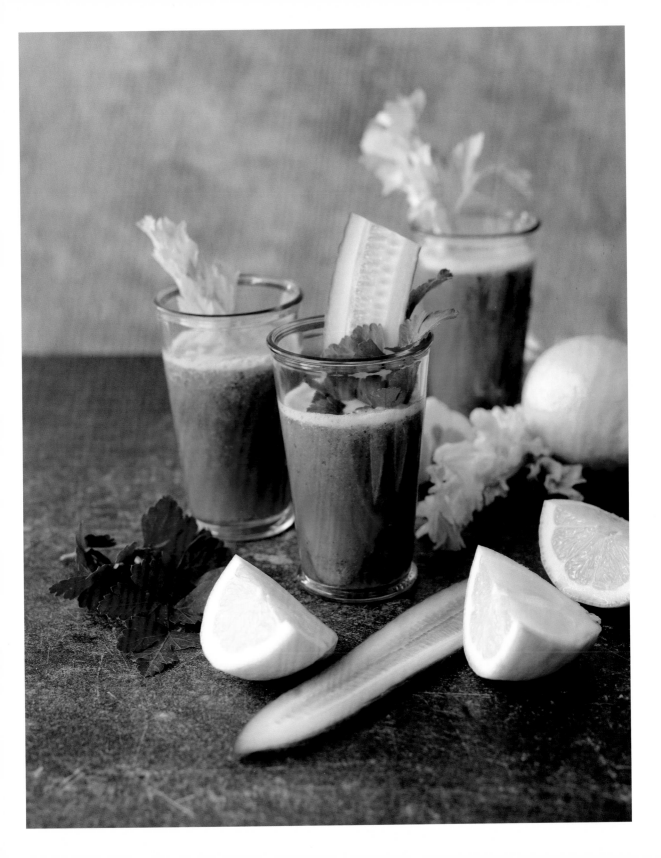

If we live like we do today—leading a sedentary lifestyle and including a lot of carbohydrates in our diet—we'll end up with constantly elevated blood sugar and lowered fat metabolism, increased stress, and heightened risk of body inflammation. Additionally, having a widely fluctuating blood sugar level will also affect our feelings of hunger and our temper. If we eat fewer carbohydrates instead, we will help our bodies to use the stored fat as energy and also reap the benefits of more even blood sugar.

Good Carbohydrates

The carbohydrates I recommend come from vegetables, fruit, and berries; greens and leaves such as arugula, spinach, iceberg lettuce, romaine, mâche, and red-leaf lettuce; and vegetables such as bell peppers, celery, asparagus, sugar snap peas, green beans, zucchini, eggplant, onions, mushrooms, cucumbers, and tomatoes.

Cruciferous vegetables like broccoli, cauliflower, white and red cabbage, fennel, and Brussels sprouts are among the best vegetables you can choose, because they're very filling and contain plenty of antioxidants. Root vegetables should be eaten sparingly, and when you do eat them, eat them in their raw state. It's also OK to eat a carrot now and then.

You can eat a small amount of berries and some fruits that don't contain a lot of carbohydrates, for example, pomegranate, rhubarb, tart apples, kiwi, and grapefruit. Try to opt for organically grown, seasonal produce as often as possible, but frozen vegetables and berries are fine also, as they sometimes contain more nutrients due to their being frozen upon harvest.

What Is Intermittent Fasting?

There are different ways to follow a fast, but, simply put, it means that during certain days or hours of the day you refrain from eating and/or just eat a limited amount of calories. In my kickstart programs, I create menus with different calorie counts for each day, and also include one or two fasting days a week, corresponding to the popular 5:2 diet. On fasting days, you'll eat approximately 500 calories, and between 1,000 and 2,000 calories on the others. To get the full effect of the fast and reap the most health benefits, it is best to minimize carbohydrates and avoid sugar altogether on fasting days.

Whichever two days you choose to fast is up to you. Many seem to prefer Mondays and Thursdays, but it is entirely flexible, and you can vary and change days as it suits you. Others fast two days in a row, like Monday and Tuesday, just to get them over and done with and to be able to enjoy the rest of the week.

Another popular diet is 16:8, which requires fasting for sixteen hours a day and eating during a period of eight hours. It means that you skip your typical breakfast meal, eat your first meal at lunch, and then finish the day eating dinner no later than 8

> **"**
>
> *To experience some hunger pangs isn't dangerous.*
>
> **"**

p.m. That way, you'll eat over a period of eight hours, between 12 p.m. and 8 p.m., and during the remaining twenty-four hours you fast by only drinking water, coffee, or tea.

You'll find both fast days and 16:8 in the Vegetarian and Raw Vegan kickstarts, but you'll find only fast days in the Detox kickstart. In the Juicing kickstart schedule, you'll find neither fast days nor 16:8, but have a consistently low calorie intake.

The Benefit of Intermittent Fasting

These days research is conducted all over world on how fasting and reduced calorie intake affect the body. I find that the most interesting studies show that the body seems to repair itself when we don't eat constantly. Much points to fasting, giving our cells an opportunity to recuperate and repair themselves, instead of being constantly busy with dividing themselves. Also shown is IGF-1 (Insulin-like Growth Factor), a growth hormone that should and does stay at a low, even level, in the same way insulin should. Elevated IGF-1 levels will put you at risk for developing ill health over time. The same applies to cholesterol and blood pressure.

What's also interesting is that blood glucose levels stabilize and remain even when we undertake short-term fasting, which suggests that we maybe shouldn't add snacks between meals to the extent we earlier believed necessary.

Intermittent fasting is relatively uncomplicated for most people to do, so it's likely that this could become a long-term solution and maybe even a lifestyle. Personally, and according to personal experience as a nutritional coach, I see more benefits to the 5:2 diet than any others that I know of. Imagine that we could fast to become healthier, to avoid having to take medications, in addition to losing excess weight or remain at a stable weight! Only the future will tell—until then you can try for yourself and see what result you achieve, whether you wish to lose weight or become healthier.

Don't You Get Hungry?

For sure your body will protest by generating hunger pangs as early as the first day you fast. But you'll probably soon realize that they're not hard to handle. Drink a cup of coffee or tea, and mineral water. Keep yourself busy and try to avoid thoughts that focus on food. You can feel safe in the knowledge that your body certainly has stored energy that it can use, and that it's not dangerous to forgo a meal or feel a hunger pang or two.

If you're still a bit unsure, take a few minutes to ponder how people coped in earlier times when food availability could vary widely from day to day. Going hungry for a few days was the norm. We are meant to survive food shortages for a few days, and not to eat constantly and as much as we do today. We didn't live on breakfast, midmorning snack, lunch, midafternoon snack, dinner, and late-night sandwich during our evolution!

To restrict oneself to 500–600 calories a day doesn't

> **"**
> *When you use different fasting practices you also force energy consumption, which speeds up metabolism.*
> **"**

equal starvation, because the body manages very well by using its reserves during these hours. That said, it is a challenge and an exciting experience with which to "tease" your brain. Your brain will, naturally, signal several times a day that it wants food—not to mention that it wants sugar! It can be quite insistent. But if you consistently answer "no," you'll win the battle after a few days. That will be noticeable. Many experience a sense of relief from sugar cravings, as well as other food urges that had earlier ruled their lives. I say it creates "food nonchalance." I just don't feel as steered to or interested in eating as before. However, my enjoyment of mealtimes is far greater when I'm actually hungry!

Can You Work Out?

Yes. Just plan your training according to fast days. A good way of combining fasting with working out is to rest on fast days and train the other days. However, you have to keep low-intensity training apart from high-intensity workouts. Low-intensity training (walking, light jogging, cycling, or yoga) on fasting days usually works very well; doing high-intensity workouts (strength training, spinning, running, or aerobics) might be a bit too taxing and tough.

Don't forget that you burn calories when you work out, and it might make you feel hungrier than you normally do on a fast day, which can add to the challenge. Get a feel for how it works for you and follow your intuition.

Increased Metabolism with Fasting

We have long believed that we need to have snacks between meals to keep our blood glucose level and to keep our metabolism running. Well, I'll assert today that this is a myth. The body works with two metabolic conditions: energy conservation and energy expenditure. The body is concentrating on storing energy for three hours after you've eaten a meal, so if you eat breakfast at 7 a.m., your body is programmed to store energy until around 10 a.m. The metabolism shifts after this (if you don't eat anything) and continues, but it's now in energy-expending mode until you eat a meal around 12 p.m., or later if you go past this time.

This means that the metabolism switches to high three hours after you have swallowed that last bite, whether you've eaten a snack or not. If you've eaten one, the body will not go into energy expenditure, but will continue in energy-savings mode, which is the exact opposite of what you're after.

When you go through different modes of fasting, you'll force your body to use energy and increase its metabolism. Another positive effect is that you stabilize your hormone balance, first of all insulin, which in turn also can contribute to better metabolism.

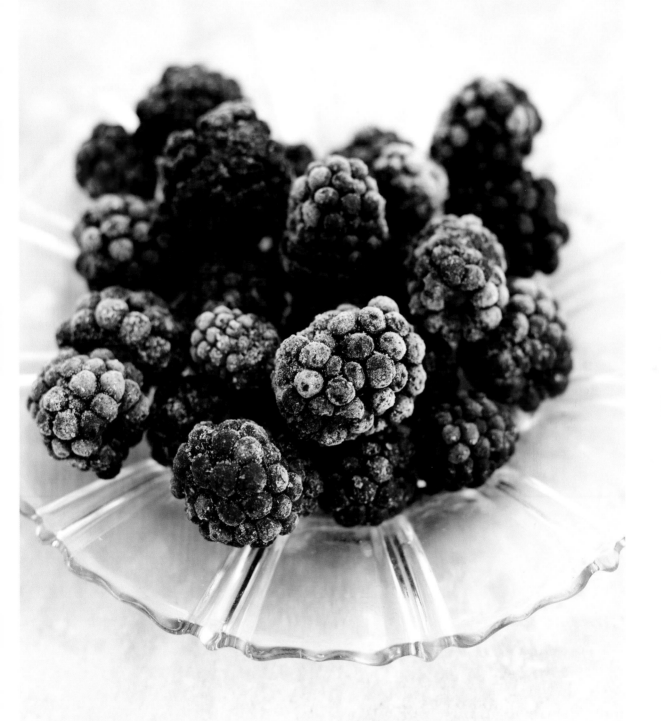

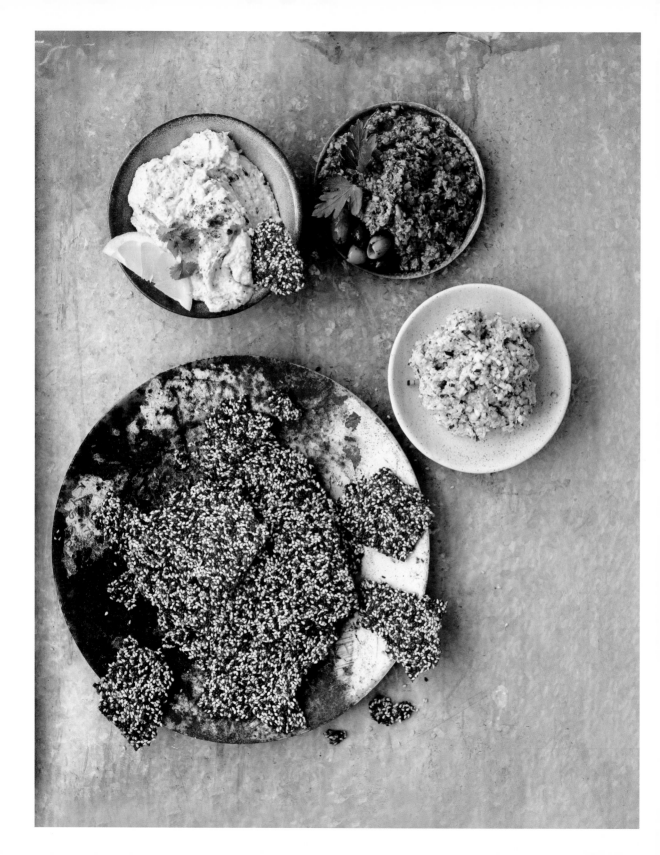

HOW TO EAT LOW CARBOHYDRATE AND VEGETARIAN

It's important to find a good replacement for animal protein. Many make the mistake of replacing meat, fish, and poultry with added pasta, rice, and lots of bread in order to feel full, and then fail to lose weight. This also adds to swings in blood glucose levels and constant cravings for sweets to replenish energy levels.

❀ Let green food fill most of your plate! Serve plenty of different filling vegetables, such as cauliflower, broccoli, white cabbage, zucchini, eggplant, fennel, and green beans.

❀ Root vegetables do contain more carbohydrates, but if they're prepared al dente the carbohydrates become slow acting. They are digested slowly and provide a nice sense of fullness. So instead of cooking and mashing them, roast carrots, beets, sweet potatoes, celeriac, and turnips in the oven.

❀ Raw foods require longer time to digest in the stomach, so they fill you up longer. They also contain more nutrients, primarily digestive enzymes. Always serve crudités (raw vegetables) with meals. Grate carrots, shred white cabbage, and enjoy raw cauliflower and broccoli now and then.

❀ Opt for vegetarian protein sources with the lowest carbohydrate content: nuts, seeds, cheese, algae, seaweed noodles, tofu, and eggs.

❀ Check the grocery store's frozen foods section for good vegetarian products like beef substitutes (Quorn or ground soy). But stay clear of those with too many additives and flour and sugar!

❀ Warm soups are more filling than you expect. It takes time for the gut to digest a vegetable soup. Two of my favorites are Tomato and Carrot Soup with Feta Cheese and Slivered Almonds (p. 173), Broccoli and Spinach Soup with Halloumi (see p. 161).

❀ Savory pies are so easily made vegetarian and with fewer carbohydrates. Nowadays there are many alternatives to white flour on the market: almond flour, buckwheat flour, coconut flour, and psyllium husk—just to name a few.

❀ To achieve a greater sense of fullness and increased protein intake, top salads and vegetables with feta cheese, goat cheese, halloumi, nuts, and seeds.

❀ Don't forget that fats are good at creating satiety—that's why I recommend that you often include, for example, olives, avocado, nuts, seeds, and oil on your plate. Try to make homemade pesto, tapenade, aioli, or a creamy mayonnaise-based dressing. This will keep you feeling full longer, and your blood glucose will stay balanced.

> *"*
> *A whole slew of scientific research*
> *points to chlorophyll's positive effect*
> *on the body.*
> *"*

Blend a Bunch of Greens—Drink a Smoothie

Greens contain lots of protein and other goodies. That's why it's an excellent idea to start making green smoothies as snacks or to serve as a meal. They're surprisingly tasty, and they keep you full for several hours. You'll need a good, strong blender for making smoothies. If your plan is to eat more vegetarian meals and make more smoothies, this is a good investment for your health.

Greens contain more precious nutrients than any other food, but all this nutrition is stored in the plants' cells. By mixing greens finely, you'll facilitate the body's uptake of all nutrients. A smoothie is also a great way of getting a larger amount of green leaves into you.

There's plenty of scientific research showing that chlorophyll has a positive effect on the body. Among other things, chlorophyll's oxygen contributes to the fight against harmful intestinal bacteria.

Did you know that plants such as nettles, clover, ground elder (also bishop's-weed), goosefoot, and dandelion contain an awful lot of nutrients, and the crowns of carrots, beets, and radishes that we often throw away have many times the nutritional value of the vegetable itself? But it's not very appetizing to make smoothies with greens, crowns, and "weeds" only, so adding some fruit and berries make them far tastier as well as more filling.

GOOD SMOOTHIE INGREDIENTS

❁ Baby spinach, regular spinach, frozen spinach, arugula, head lettuce, bok choy, endives, kale, Swiss chard.
❁ Crowns from radishes, carrots, and beets.
❁ Plants like nettles, clover, dandelion, and lamb's quarters.
❁ Fresh green herbs such as basil, oregano, thyme, chervil, chives, rosemary, and dill weed.
❁ All cruciferous vegetables like broccoli, Brussels sprouts, savoy cabbage, pointed cabbage, and cauliflower.
❁ A bunch of other vegetables: sugar snap peas, frozen peas, green beans, asparagus, green bell pepper, leeks, zucchini, avocado, sprouts, cucumber, and celery.

Mix the above with:

❁ Kiwi, mango, banana, pineapple, melon, orange, all types of berries, lime, and lemon.
❁ By all means add some cinnamon, ginger, garlic, chili, sweet almonds, and/or ice cubes, if you like.

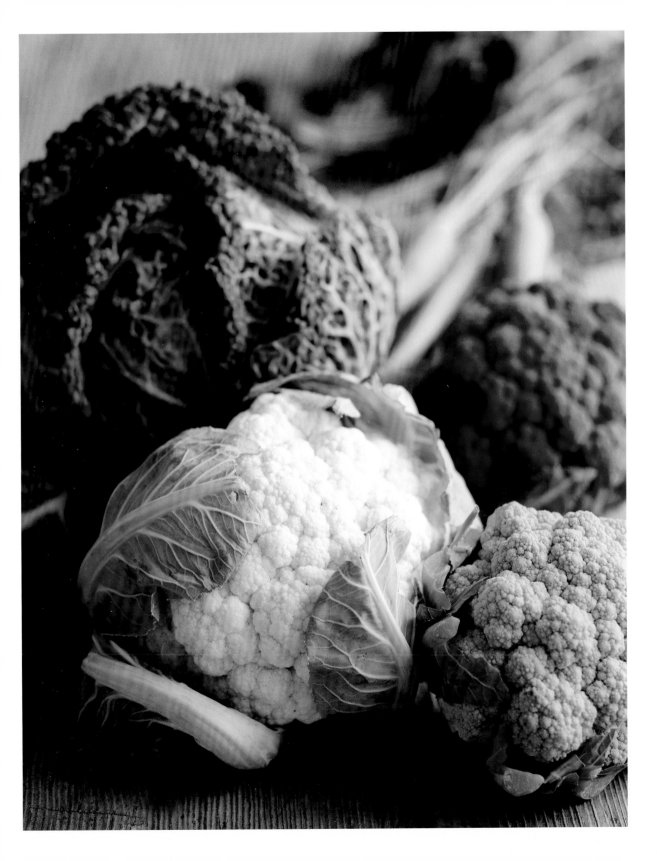

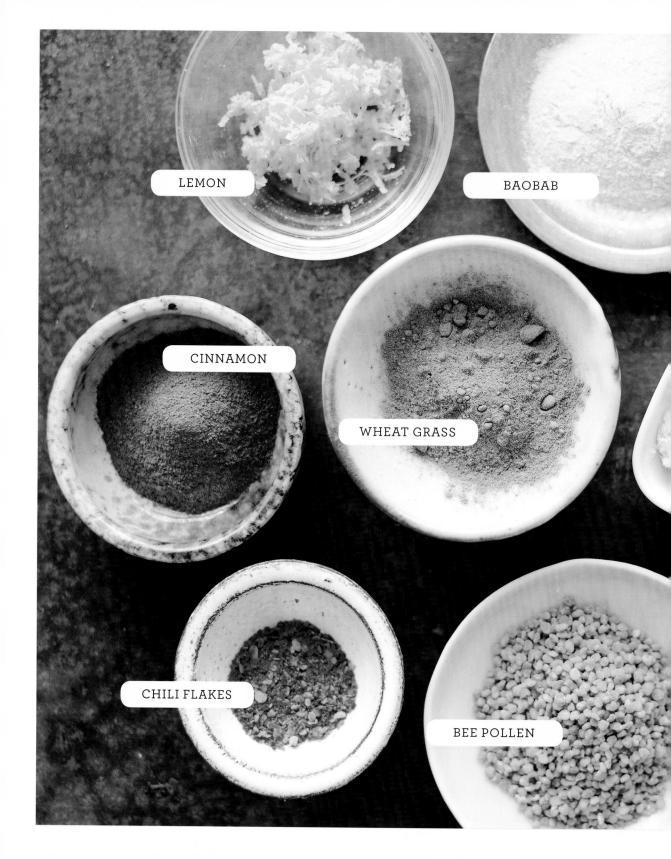

LEMON

BAOBAB

CINNAMON

WHEAT GRASS

CHILI FLAKES

BEE POLLEN

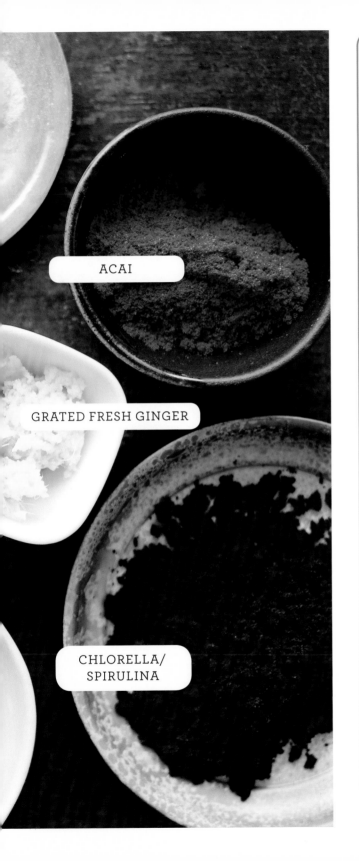

ACAI

GRATED FRESH GINGER

CHLORELLA/
SPIRULINA

NATURAL BOOSTS

There are many raw ingredients that can strengthen your body and also provide you with more energy. Below I have listed some ingredients that you're allowed to include in your beverages and dishes.

Lemon is cleansing and contains lots of vitamin C. Preferably drink a large glass of lemon water (see p. 107) every morning.

Baobab (powder) comes from tree fruits filled with fiber, vitamin C, magnesium, and calcium.

Acai (powder) is from a dark lilac berry packed with antioxidant anthocyanin; it is rich in vitamins and omega-9 fatty acids.

Cinnamon is excellent for blood glucose, digestion, and the circulatory system.

Wheatgrass (powder) is dried wheatgrass and contains 70 percent chlorophyll. Cleanses and strengthens the blood and the body through inclusion of plenty of different minerals, vitamins, and amino acids. One dose is the equivalent of 2½ pounds (1 kg) of vegetables.

Ginger cleanses and gets rid of toxins and strengthens your immune system.

Cayenne pepper/chili is an expectorant and is good for the circulatory system and metabolism.

Bee pollen contains about 205 bioactive substances, 16 vitamins, 27 minerals, and 22 amino acids. They are small vitamin bombs, for sure!

Chlorella/spirulina are microalgae crammed with chlorophyll, vitamins, and minerals. They have a cleansing effect.

Other boosting raw ingredients:
Camu camu, turmeric, hawthorn, and lucuma.

TIME TO SET A GOAL

I will provide you with ready-made diet meal schedules, but it is up to you to do the work. Now the time has come to set a goal! What do you want it to be?

Once you know what your objective is, you can actively work at it so it becomes reality. It's not until you start imagining your future aim—how you want it to look—that you can seriously work to affect your present situation.

An objective is a result you wish to achieve; it is a tangible picture of your desired goal. An objective is *not* what you do to reach this end result. An objective has to be a desired goal, not an activity.

When you decide to do something, when you have decided that this is the way it is going to be—that's when you take control over your actions, and why you do them. As the objective is something you want to reach and something you look forward to, it will also give you energy and motivation.

THREE POINTS FOR SETTING A GOAL

Today's situation—where are you today?

_____

_____

_____

_____

Desired situation—what is your goal?

_____

_____

_____

_____

The road to the goal—what do you need to do to reach your goal? Which kickstart suits you?

_____

_____

_____

_____

Become Your Own Coach

Some days it's difficult to feel motivated. Everything feels heavy, the body protests, and you're cold, tired, weak, full of cravings, angry, irritated, restless, and out of patience. These are common symptoms for anyone starting a new nutritional plan, because it might be a significant change to lay off sugar and simultaneously remove all fast-acting carbohydrates that usually provide quick energy boosts.

It might take a few days for your body to get used to new foods. Different reactions and feelings might emerge, but they often disappear after about a week, because the body is getting used to the new rules and gets its energy from the diet schedule you're following. You will have to get through these first days, this phase, for it to become easier later on.

When things start to feel really heavy and cumbersome, remind yourself why you want to make changes to your health and remember that what you do is well worth it!

Three Mainstays That Will Help You Reach Your Goal

There are three important aspects to keep in mind when starting your new daily lifestyle. These are: *motivation*, *planning*, and *self-discipline*.

You can look at these pillars as a stool with three legs, and you need to stay focused on all three legs for the stool to stand or for you to succeed. If you start to ignore one of the legs, the stool will tip over, and your ability to reach your objective will be negatively affected.

You'll get lots of help with **Motivation** through the information contained in this book, with plenty of tasty and easy-to-prepare recipes and handsome pictures to inspire you. Of course, you must also work at motivating yourself—for example, find enjoyment in preparing the evening meal, or become interested in heal-thy, alternative pursuits. If you just walk around feeling sorry for yourself and only count the days and hours until the whole schedule is finished, motivation will wane. Think positive! Start your schedule with passion and interest, and things will go so much smoother. Tips to boost motivation: Leave a piece of clothing you want to be able to wear in a month's time within view. Each day, think how much further along you are in your goal to be able to fit into it. Or, pin up a picture of yourself when you felt happy with your weight and body.

Planning is critical to success. I mean planning the whole way. Many are very good at planning in the early stages, but forget to keep it up later on. Don't make this mistake! Decide here and now that you will plan your food and workouts for each week, and note it down. To your personal kickstart add your weight and measurements for the duration of the plan—even if they don't change as fast as you would like, or if you've cheated a little. Just get it down on paper and get back on the wagon.

Practicing **Self-discipline** is the most difficult task of the three, and presents the biggest challenge. Some people are born with it, while others have to work more at it. In this respect the book will be of little help, and you really have to work with yourself. Carefully follow your plans—for example, if you have penciled in a 45-minute walk for Wednesday evening, you can't sink into the couch instead because it's raining. Our brain is very crafty and finds many reasons to cheat and conveniently "forget" things, and that's when self-discipline needs to step in and save the situation!

A tip for putting a stop to things when focus and self-discipline are slipping is to use the two-minute rule. This means that, for example, if you feel that you just *must* buy that pastry, stop your thought there and then, and look at your watch. Talk yourself down for two minutes and remind yourself that pastries have no place in the diet schedule, and that it is not a smart move to eat one! Two minutes are a great opportunity to change your mind-set to another and better one.

The same applies when your brain tells you that you're too tired to go to the gym or to take a walk. Check your watch and reason with yourself for two minutes about the pros and cons of sidestepping the plan, about the short-term relief compared to the long-term benefits. My guess is that you'll realize that the long-term benefits are more important. Try this rule and experience what a positive and strong effect it can have on you.

Other Benefits of Nutritional Planning

This list can be made much longer, and naturally it's very personal how you experience changes. But the usual comments I hear are:

- feeling much better mentally
- feeling more energized and having much more energy during the day
- sleeping much better
- no cravings for candy
- much better digestion
- the great feeling that comes from eating healthy and working out
- feeling happier and being more even-tempered
- enjoying the new foods and having an improved taste sense
- feeling healthier and not catching colds as frequently as before
- enjoying shopping for new clothes
- taking an interest in trying out new sports and enjoying being active
- feeling lighter and slimmer

Coach Yourself for 10 Minutes

Read through and answer the questions below. Take the time to think through how you feel and how you experience your current situation and what you would like to change about it. What you write down is important in your work of self-coaching and to reach the objective you have decided on. Remind yourself *each and every day* why you're working for this change, and feel enjoyment when you reflect on your future journey through these coming weeks!

How do you want to feel when you have reached your goal?

_____

_____

_____

What is your biggest obstacle?

_____

_____

_____

What can you do to overcome this obstacle?

_____

_____

_____

Imagine how you feel after you've finished a two-week kickstart:

What do you look like? _____

_____

How do you feel? _____

_____

_____

How have you evolved? _____

_____

_____

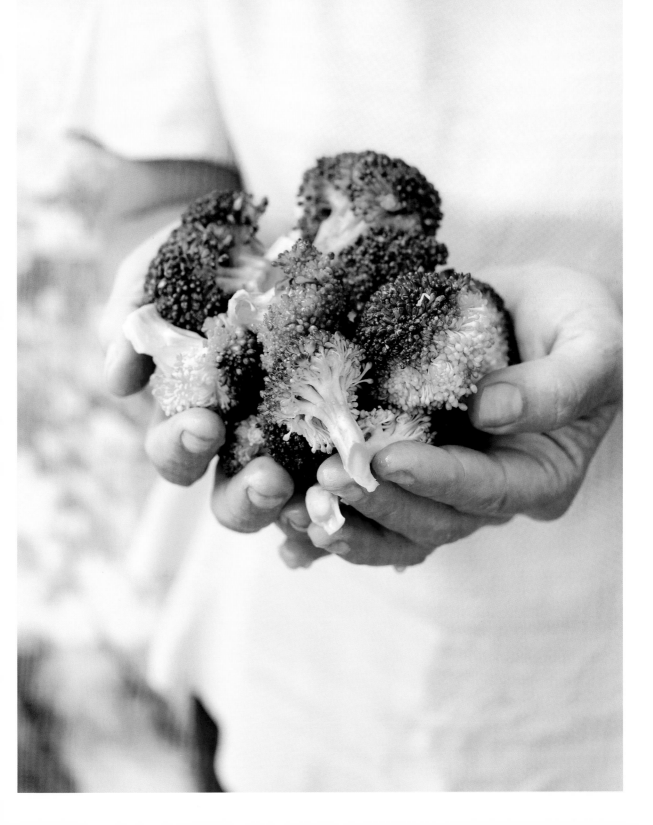

SOME THOUGHTS AND ADVICE ABOUT WEIGHT LOSS

Sometimes it can be difficult to get your metabolism and weight loss going. Many factors can play a part in this. After all my years as a nutritional adviser, I have realized that in these cases only patience works. Give your body the opportunity to feel comfortable with its new nutritional diet. Continue even if you haven't lost a lot of weight. Don't give up! Don't forget to check your body measurements regularly to see if something has happened—sometimes you'll notice changes there first, before the scales.

Many times a weight problem can have a genetic component, which means that you have to fight more than others to keep off excess weight. Other reasons might be:

You Have Yo-Yo Dieted Frequently
Maybe you've gone through cycles when you've lived on meal replacements such as shakes and soups, or perhaps followed a bananas or cabbage soup method or some other odd diet. Then you have to allow your body to repair the damage. The prerequisite to allowing this to happen is a diet of fresh and natural foods with good fats, proteins, and plenty of vegetables. A variable daily calorie intake will also kickstart your metabolism.

You Feel Stressed Out
Stress and sleep are important factors when it comes to weight loss success. Do you have too many "must-dos" and are you too busy at work or at home? Are you a worrier and do you sleep badly? Cortisol, a stress hormone, is secreted, which provides more energy by elevating blood glucose, which in turn raises insulin secretion. As a result, the body stores fat (see p. 10), so it becomes even more important to do what you can to deal with excessive stress, and to make sure that you get enough sleep if you have a weight problem.

You Can't Tolerate Certain Foods
Some people have difficulty digesting milk proteins and milk sugars (lactose), which could cause problems with weight loss. Dairy products can also have a negative effect on weight, as they promote the release of extra insulin. This might make you feel bloated, and can cause digestive problems. Try eliminating cream, crème fraîche, yogurt, cheese, and other dairy products (not butter, though) for a week and see how this comes up on the scales.

The same applies to nuts. If eliminating dairy products doesn't help, try forgoing nuts instead, and see if this makes it better.

Your Hormones Are at Fault
There are more than 50 different types of hormones in the human body, including insulin, cortisol, adrenaline, noradrenaline, serotonin, dopamine, endorphins, oxytocin, estrogen, testosterone, and progesterone.

Hormonal imbalance is a common and increasing problem—primarily among women. You can also have a slow metabolism due to an underactive thyroid. Metabolism can be tested with a simple blood test at your nearest clinic, and the remedy is usually a supplement in the form of tablets.

Estrogen levels in women and testosterone levels in men decrease in the change of life, and this can add a few pounds. The risk of having a hormonal imbalance is greater if you have lived on refined carbohydrates over a long period of time, are stressed out, get too little sleep, and are sedentary. It might take a long time to rectify this imbalance, but it can be done. Follow the diet schedule, and have patience!

SOME THOUGHTS AND ADVICE ABOUT THE SCALES

Weigh Yourself Once a Week

I recommend that you choose a specific day to weigh yourself, and why not make it Monday? You may get the wrong picture of your true weight if you weigh yourself more often. Many factors influence weight, such as if you have your period, if you haven't been to the toilet, or what you have eaten or drunk during the day.

Weigh Yourself at the Same Time Every Week

Your weight can vary up to 4½–5 pounds (2½ kg) between morning and evening. Weigh yourself at the same time each week, preferably in the morning after you have been to the toilet—and preferably without clothes.

Take Bodily Measurements

You will often see results earlier on the tape measure than on the scales. Measure yourself once a week at the same time as your weigh-in, and check what has happened. For some, the result is more visible on the tape measure, while for others it is on the scales. There's nothing strange in this, since we're all different. Never compare yourself to anybody else.

Be Kind to Yourself

In order to not be disappointed, "cushion" your goal weight. If your goal weight is 143½ pounds (65 kg), but the scales still show 150 pounds (68 kg), feel happy anyway! As I've said before, the day's activities might influence the scales, and, if you're female, you're more likely gain water weight at certain times. Give yourself a pat on the back for making this weight journey instead of feeling disappointed.

The Number on the Scales Doesn't Tell the Whole Story

The numbers on the scales are not what are most important. Don't forget all the other health benefits you acquire by eating according to your kickstart menu schedule. Perhaps your gut feels better, you have more energy, you sleep better, you have more balanced blood glucose, and you feel less cravings for sweets. These are benefits that can feel just as valuable as a weight loss.

"

Weigh yourself once a week. Weigh yourself at the same time each week. Check your body measurements. Be kind to yourself. And remember: the numbers on the scales don't tell the whole story.

"

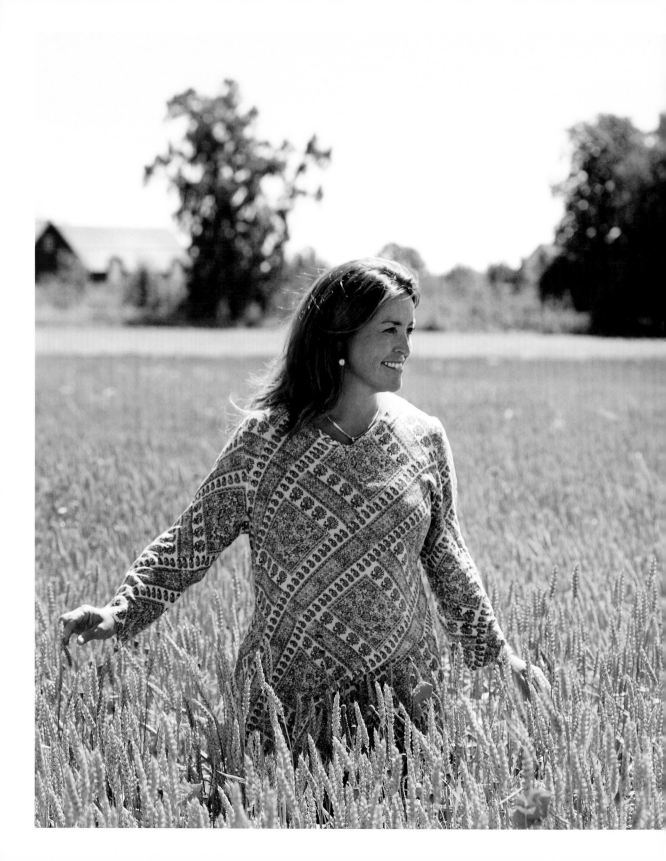

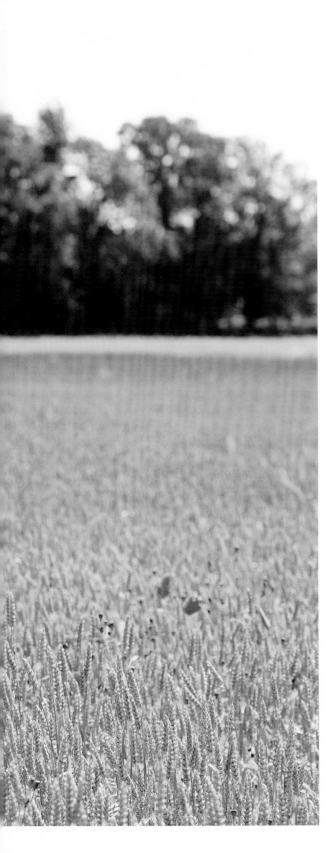

A Lifestyle for You

Everything is about finding the lifestyle that works for you. I have to work at it myself every day—it isn't something that happens automatically.

Don't be too hard on yourself. Sometimes we veer off track, but it's all about getting back on track again immediately, and keep going. I usually say that a year has 365 days, and if we get it right during three hundred of them, we still have sixty-five during which we can be a bit more forgiving.

I coach lots of people who have decided to make a life change, on a daily basis. I do it through my online classes, which you can find at www.ulrikaskickstart.se. I hope to see you in one of my classes!

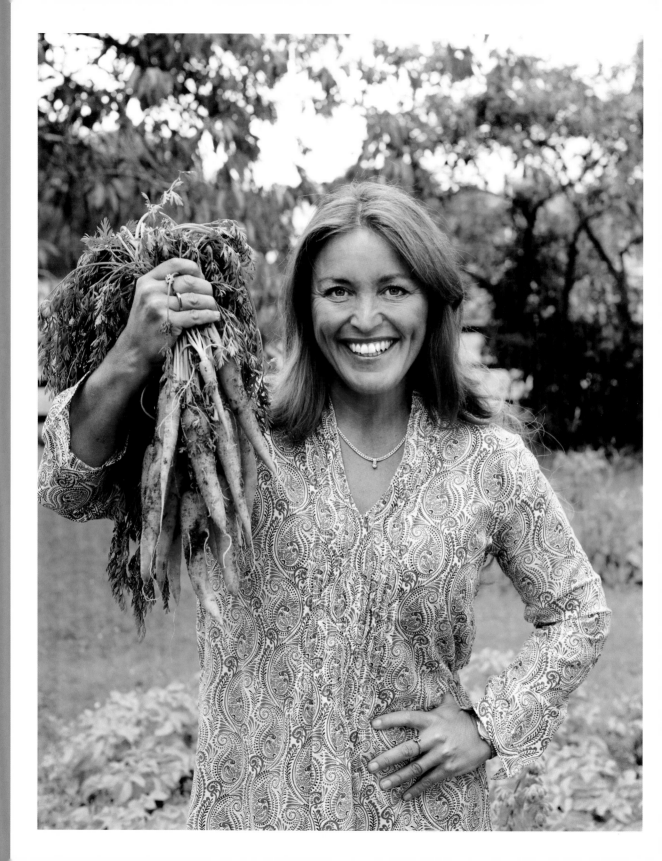

– KICKSTART –
DETOX
– RECIPES AND MEAL SCHEDULE –

I usually recommend that everyone do a detox cure/kickstart twice a year, and it should last at least fourteen days—better yet, twenty-eight days. The cure has clear and tangible effects for the body that also last a long time. It is impossible to achieve the same effect in just a few days.

It is a fact that the first days of a detox cure are a challenge for the body's cleansing organs, as they have to work full-time to break down toxins and waste products that have collected in the body. There's also many of what we call free radicals in circulation, and that might make you more prone to experiencing flu-like symptoms, for example, or you feel chilled and tired.

These negative feelings will be gone in about four or five days and be replaced by energy, making the remainder of your days of detox—pardon the pun—pure pleasure!

A complete detox cure is like a vacation for the body. All the organs function better, and you become familiar with which foods are good for you. You might also find out that certain regular foods aren't especially important, and perhaps you don't even feel good after consuming them. Many find this out about dairy products and gluten.

This is a sign for those who of you have lived with pain, gut and digestive problems, bad sleep patterns, and a stressed-out body for many years (and now realize how much better you feel), that it is time for the sake of your health to change your nutrition for the long term.

We can liken the detox cure to pressing the alt+ctrl+del on the computer. These are the buttons you frantically press to reboot your computer when its screen freezes, hoping everything goes back to normal. The same thing happens in the detox cure—the body is cleaned from the inside out; it reboots and begins to function well again and doesn't "freeze" quite so often. For some, the detox cure is revolutionary, and they want to keep going longer than fourteen days. There is nothing stopping anyone from doing so.

You'll decrease the amount of food you eat during the detox cure, but you will still feel satisfied. You will eat mostly natural carbohydrates and natural fats. You'll eat a relatively small portion of protein to allow the liver to focus on breaking down toxins and waste products in your body.

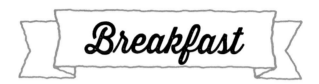

Tasty breakfasts that barely affect your blood glucose, while leaving you feeling pleasantly full. This makes it far easier for you to keep to your meal schedule.

KALE SMOOTHIE

A filling smoothie brimming with the antioxidant chlorophyll.

83 CALORIES/SERVES 2

2⅔ ounces (75 g) kale, coarsely chopped
½ apple, core and seeds removed
1 stalk celery
3⅓ ounces (1 dl) frozen pineapple pieces
6¾ fluid ounces (2 dl) water
3⅓ fluid ounces (1 dl) oat milk

1. Place the kale in a blender.
2. Slice the apple and celery and add to the blender with the pineapple pieces.
3. Add water and oat milk, and blend into a smoothie.

SOY YOGURT WITH CITRUS AND PISTACHIOS

You can use a variety of other fruits and nuts.

244 CALORIES/SERVES 1

½ grapefruit
½ blood orange
3⅓ fluid ounces plain soy yogurt
2 tablespoons pistachios, chopped

1. Cut off the citrus peel, and slice or cut the fruit into segments.
2. Place the fruit in a bowl and dot with the yogurt.
3. Top with the chopped pistachios.

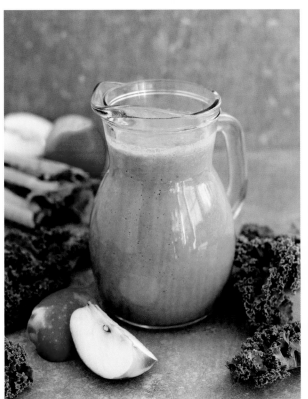

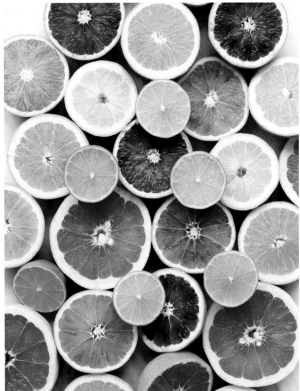

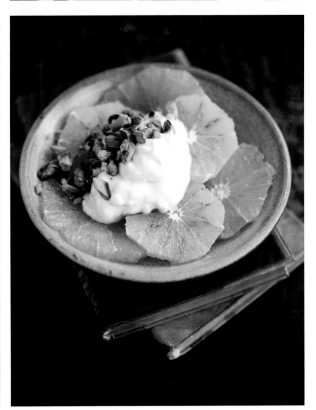

"
*Tasty and fresh
starts to the day.*

"

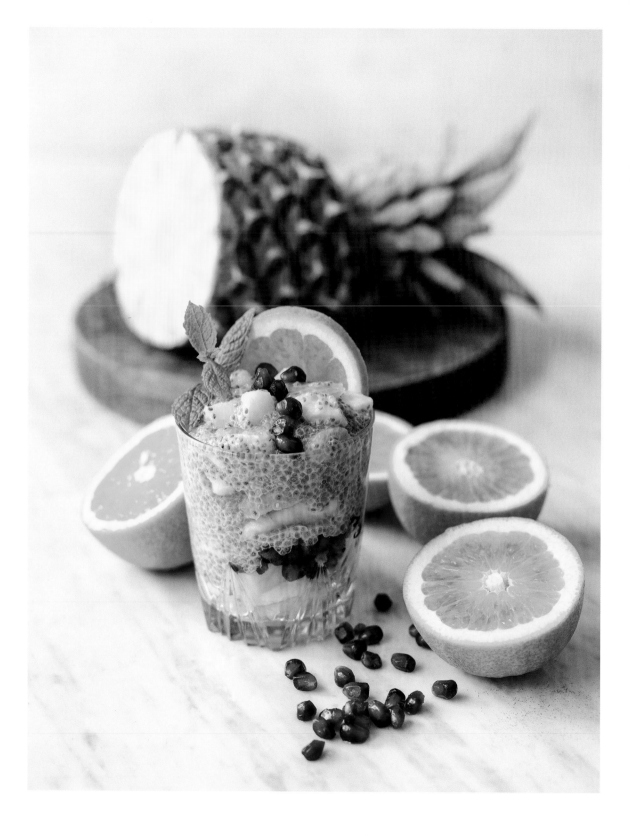

Chia Seed Porridge

Gluten-free porridge from a small seed called chia. Add in flavor with fruit or berries, and mix with almond milk and vanilla. Delicious!

269 CALORIES/SERVES 1

2 tablespoons chia seeds
5 fluid ounces (1½ dl) almond milk
1 pinch vanilla powder
1 orange
½ cup (1 dl) chopped fresh pineapple

Topping

Seeds from ½ pomegranate, for garnish
Sprig of mint, for garnish
Slice of orange, for garnish

1. Mix chia seeds and almond milk in a bowl. Stir in the vanilla powder and let the mixture sit for 30 minutes or overnight.
2. Dilute the porridge with more milk if needed. Cut off the orange peel with a sharp knife and slice the orange in fine segments. Cut the segments into smaller pieces and stir them into the porridge together with the chopped pineapple.
3. Scoop the porridge into a glass bowl and garnish with pomegranate seeds, a sprig of mint, and an orange slice.

Quinoa Granola
WITH HONEY-ROASTED WALNUTS

Gluten-free granola that takes all of five minutes to prepare! Quinoa puffs can be found on the grocery store's health food shelves or in well-stocked health food stores.

175 CALORIES/(1 SERVING = 4 TABLESPOONS) – **MAKES APPROXIMATELY 15 SERVINGS**

2 cups (5 dl) quinoa puffs
6¾ ounces (2 dl) almonds
3⅓ ounces (1 dl) pistachios
6¾ ounces (2 dl) yellow raisins
1¾ ounces (½ dl) freeze-dried blueberries

Honey-Roasted Walnuts

6¾ ounces (2 dl) chopped walnuts
1 tablespoon honey

1. Mix all the ingredients except walnuts and honey in a bowl.
2. Heat up a skillet and roast the walnuts until they are slightly colored, stirring continuously.
3. Drizzle with the honey and stir it in.
4. Set the skillet aside and let the nuts cool down, and then mix them into the granola. Store the granola in a jar with a tight-fitting lid.

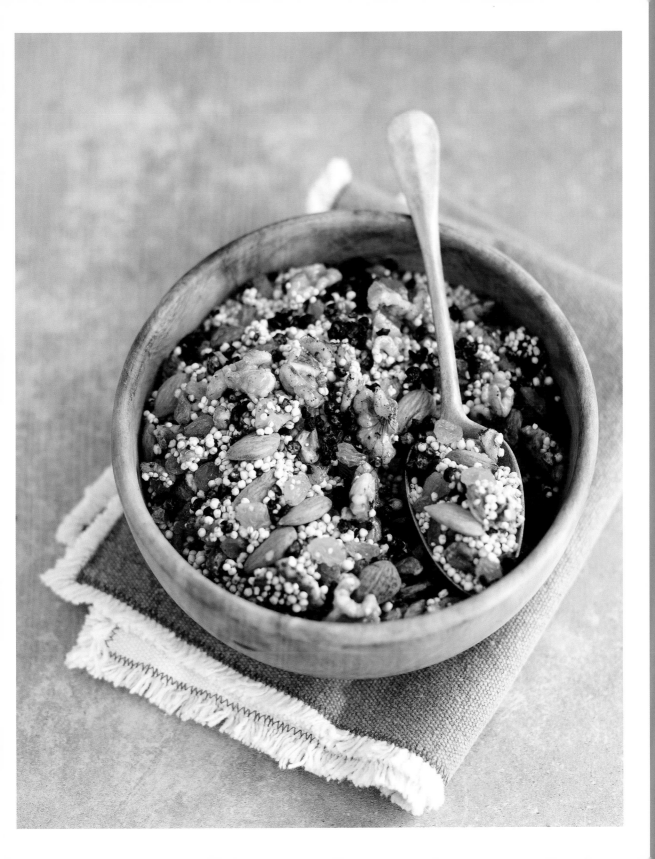

Sesame Seed Crackers

A truly tasty crispbread for breakfast or as a snack.

SESAME SEED CRACKERS

32 CALORIES/PIECE – MAKES APPROXIMATELY 20 PIECES

6¾ ounces (2 dl) white sesame seeds
3⅓ ounces (1 dl) black sesame seeds
1¾ ounces (½ dl) chia seeds
3⅓ ounces (1 dl) corn flour
½ teaspoon salt
1¾ fluid ounces (½ dl) canola oil
6¾ fluid ounces boiling water

1. Preheat the oven to 300°F (150°C). In a bowl, mix all ingredients to make a batter.
2. Spread the batter out on a baking sheet lined with parchment paper.
3. Place another piece of parchment paper on top, and spread out the batter until it forms a thin layer that covers most of the baking sheet. Remove the top piece of parchment paper.
4. Bake the cracker in the oven for about 1 hour. Let it cool and then break it into pieces.

SESAME SEED CRACKERS WITH PECORINO CHEESE

260 CALORIES/SERVES 1

5 cherry tomatoes—still attached to the branch
2 slices pecorino cheese
2 sesame seed crackers
Some pea shoots, for garnish

1. Slice the cherry tomatoes.
2. Place the slices of pecorino on the crackers and top with tomatoes and pea shoots.

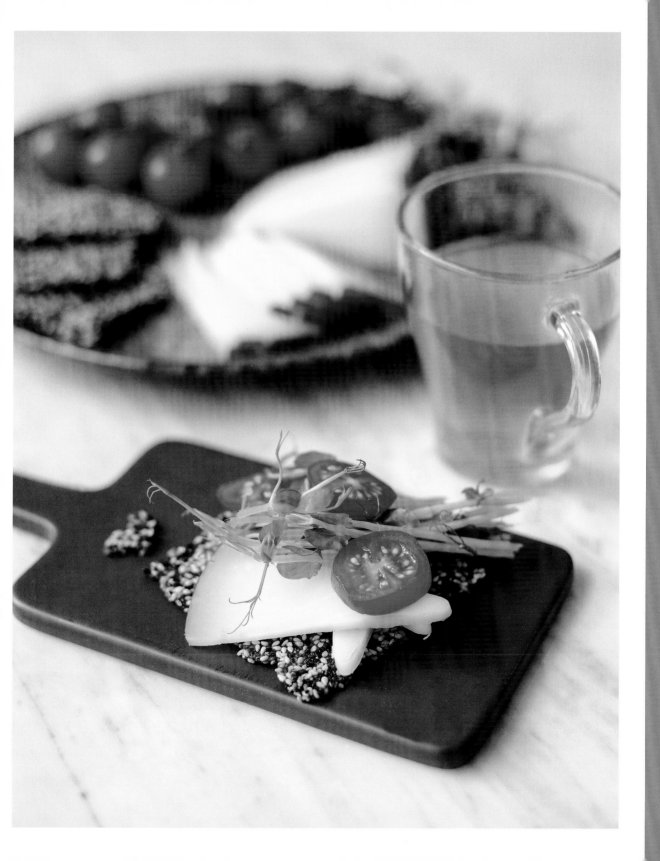

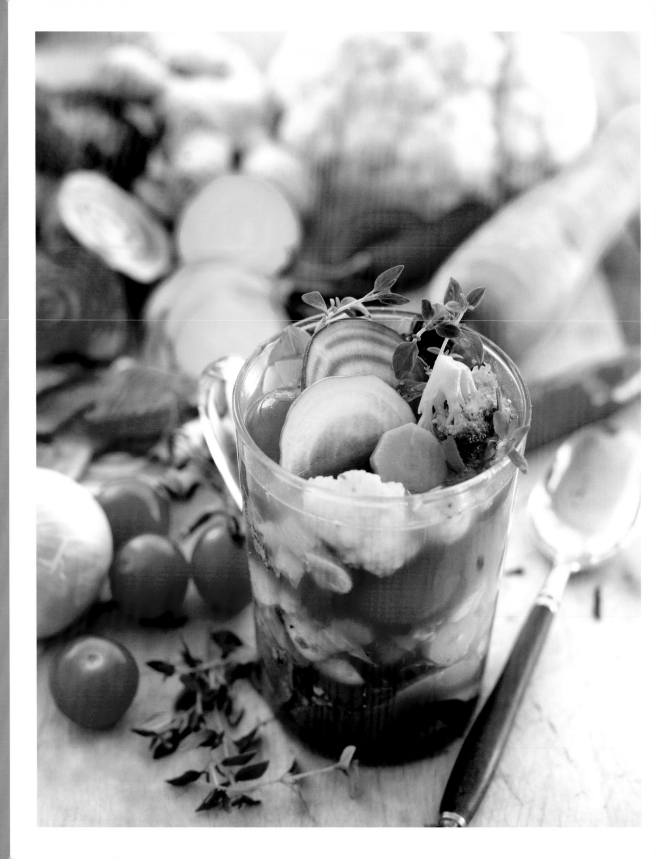

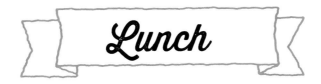

Detox Soup

A satisfying soup full of crisp vegetables.

150 CALORIES/SERVING. – **SERVES 2**

½ small cauliflower
½ small broccoli stem and florets
1 carrot
10 mushrooms
½ yellow onion
1 teaspoon olive oil
1 clove garlic, grated
1 tablespoon fresh ginger, grated
½ small red chili, finely chopped
⅓ teaspoon turmeric
Salt
Black pepper
2⅓ cups (6 dl) water
1 cube vegetable stock
Approximately ¾ ounce
  (20 g) fresh spinach leaves

Decoration

Fresh thyme for garnish
3½ ounces (100 g) cherry
  tomatoes
Slices of different types of beets
  for garnish, optional

1. Cut the vegetables into smaller pieces. Heat oil in a large pot and add in all the vegetables. Mix in the garlic, ginger, chili, and turmeric, and sauté for a minute or two. Season with salt and pepper.

2. Add the water and stock cube. Bring to a boil and let it simmer over low heat for about 10 minutes.

3. Stir in the spinach and cherry tomatoes (if using) just before serving. Pour into large cups or into bowls, and garnish with thyme and sliced beets, if desired.

Rice Wraps
WITH MANGO AND CURRY SAUCE

Rice papers are practical and fun to use for wraps. You'll find them in the Asian food section at your grocery store. You can easily vary this recipe using other vegetables and dips.

200 CALORIES/SERVING. – SERVES 4

Mango and Curry Sauce

3⅓ ounces (1 dl) plain cashews
1 mango
Juice of ½ lime
A few mint leaves
1 tablespoon curry powder
½ tablespoon turmeric

Rice Wraps

2 carrots
5¼ ounces (150 g) fresh sugar snap peas
4 stalks celery
10 rice papers
3⅓ ounces (1 dl) white cabbage, slivered
3½ ounces (1 dl) red cabbage, slivered

1. Start with the mango and curry sauce. Let the cashews soak in water for 8 hours, and then drain the nuts thoroughly.
2. Peel the mango and remove the pit. Cut the mango into pieces and place them in a food processor with the drained cashews and the rest of the sauce ingredients. Blend into a smooth sauce and pour it into a bowl.
3. Cut the carrots into thin sticks. Julienne the sugar snap peas and the celery into thin strips.
4. Soak a piece of rice paper in a plate filled with cold water. When the paper has softened (approximately 20 seconds) set it on a cutting board. Place a bit of all the chopped vegetables in the middle of the paper and roll it into wrap. Repeat with the rest of the rice papers.
5. Cut the wraps in half and place them on a serving dish. Serve with the sauce.

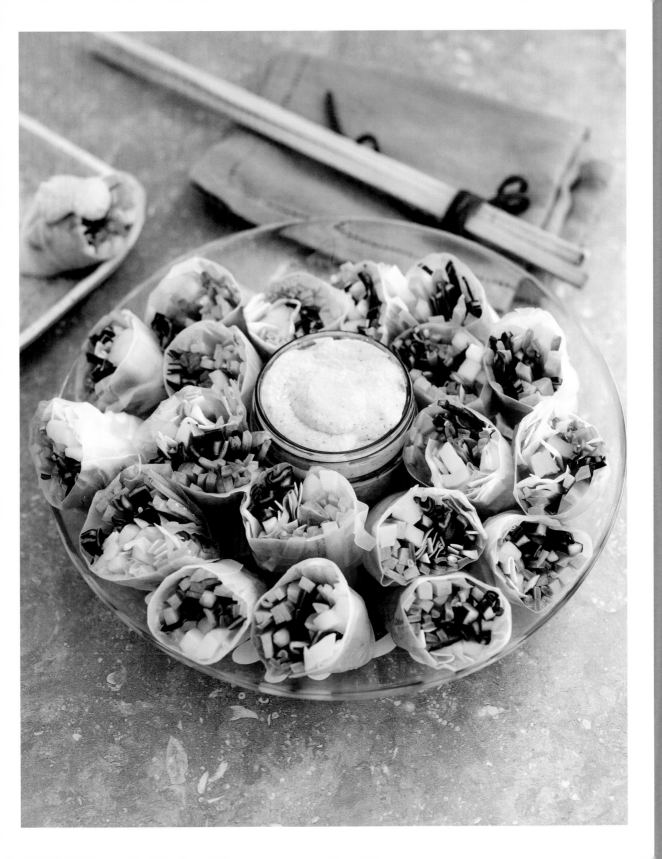

Vegetables
WITH HUMMUS DIP

*Would you prefer some other vegetables than those I've suggested? No problem.
Choose your favorite vegetables and dip them in this tasty hummus.*

435 CALORIES–SERVES 1

½ **red bell pepper**
½ **green bell pepper**
1 **celery stalk**
1 **carrot**
6 **radishes**
1¾ **fluid ounces (½ dl)**
 hummus

Hummus

1 **can (14 ounces or**
 400 g) chickpeas
1 **clove garlic, coarsely**
 chopped
½ **bunch of fresh**
 cilantro
1 **tablespoon sesame oil**
1¾ **fluid ounces (½ dl)**
 olive oil
Juice of ½ lemon
Salt
Black pepper

1. Cut the vegetables into sticks and place them on a platter.
2. Drain the chickpeas in a strainer. Rinse with cold water and let drain. Place the chickpeas in a food processor along with the rest of the hummus ingredients and process to a smooth mixture. Season with salt and pepper, and add more lemon juice if desired.
3. Serve the hummus with the vegetable sticks.

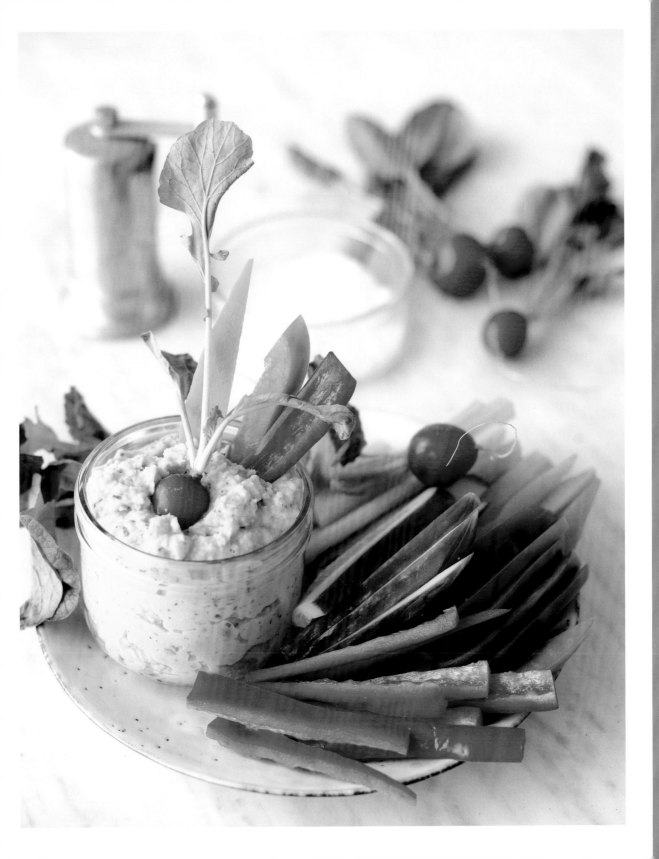

BELL PEPPER AND
Feta Cheese Gratin

*Oven-baked bell peppers are delicious and easy to make for dinner.
But these stuffed bell peppers are equally perfect as a snack.*

291 CALORIES/SERVES 4

6 yellow bell peppers (try pointy ones such as Pequillos)

5¼ ounces (150 g) feta cheese

1¾ fluid ounces (½ dl) ajvar roasted pepper relish

2¼ ounces (65 g) arugula

1¾ fluid ounce (½ dl) green pesto (see p. 58, or use store-bought pesto)

Salt

Black pepper

Seeds of ½ pomegranate, for garnish

1. Preheat the oven to 437°F (225°C). Halve the peppers lengthwise and remove the centers.
2. Fill the pepper halves with crumbled feta cheese and ajvar relish. Place the peppers on a parchment-lined baking sheet and leave them in the oven for about 15 to 20 minutes.
3. Scatter arugula over a serving platter and place the pepper halves on top.
4. Dollop the pepper halves with green pesto and season with salt and pepper. Garnish with pomegranate seeds.

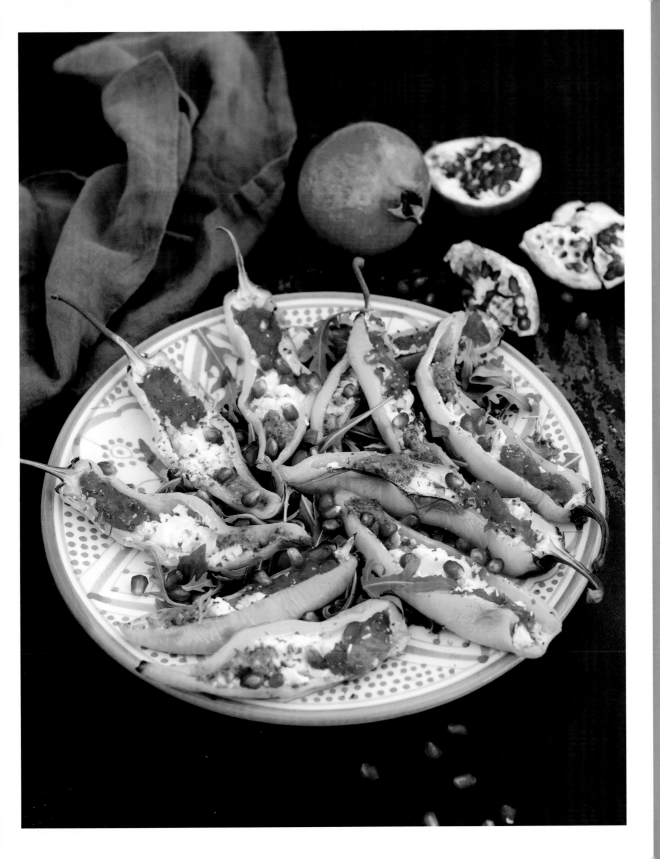

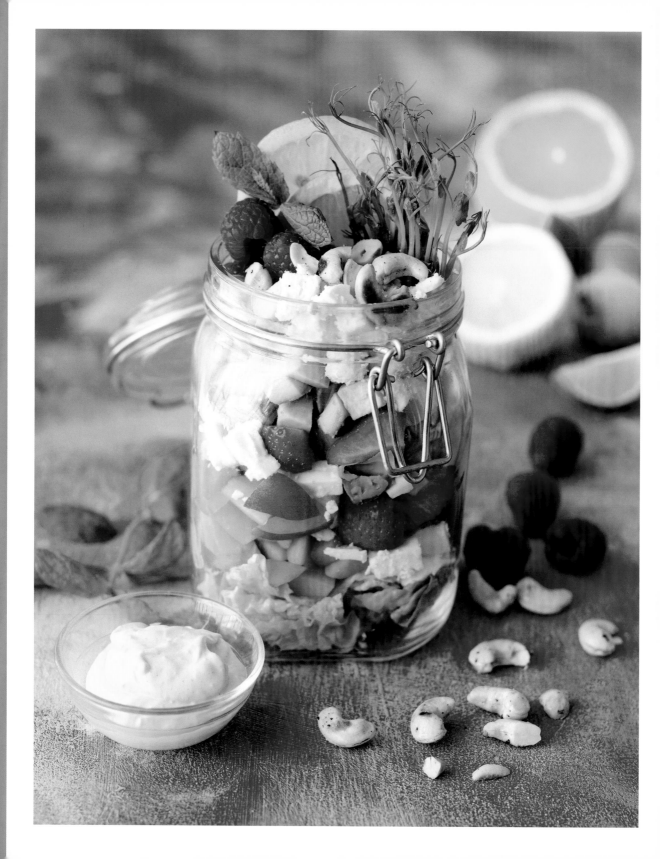

FRUITY FETA CHEESE SALAD
in a Jar

Why relegate salad to a plastic container when we can fill attractive glass jars instead? Build your own salad using fruit, berries, cheese, and nuts. Then stir together in a bowl with saffron aioli made with mayonnaise, salt, pepper, and a small pinch of saffron—or buy it ready-made.

690 CALORIES/SERVES 1

1 head lettuce

3 fresh apricots

2⅔ ounces (80 g) feta cheese, divided

5 strawberries

½ avocado

5 raspberries

1⅔ ounces (½ dl) roasted cashews seasoned with black pepper

Pea shoots, for garnish

Orange slices, for garnish

Lemon slices, for garnish

1 sprig fresh mint, for garnish

4 tablespoons saffron aioli

1. Chop the lettuce and place it in a glass jar.
2. Slice the apricots and sprinkle them over the lettuce. Crumble half of the feta cheese into the jar. Slice the strawberries and put them on top of the cheese.
3. Dice the avocado and sprinkle it on top of the strawberries. Crumble and add in the remaining feta cheese. Finish layering with the raspberries and the roasted cashews.
4. Garnish with pea shoots, orange slices, lemon slices, and fresh mint. Serve with saffron aioli.

Beet Quinoa
WITH FETA CHEESE

This is one of my favorite dishes. The white quinoa is colored red when it is mixed with the cooked beets. Beautiful yes, but first and foremost absolutely delicious!

520 CALORIES/SERVES 4

6¾ ounces (2 dl) quinoa

3 beets, cooked and peeled

3½ ounces (100 g) soybeans

1 tablespoon olive oil

1 teaspoon red wine vinegar

2 tablespoons parsley, chopped

Salt

Black pepper

2¼ ounces (65 g) arugula

5¼ ounces (150 g) feta cheese

½ red onion, julienned

1¾ ounce (50 g) pecans, coarsely chopped

Parsley, for garnish

Grapefruit segments, for garnish

1. Cook the quinoa according to the directions on the packet, approximately 13 minutes. Drain off the water.
2. Cut the beets into small dice and place them in a bowl. Add the quinoa, soybeans, oil, vinegar, and parsley. Season with salt and pepper.
3. Divide the arugula between the plates and place the beet quinoa on top. Crumble with feta cheese and garnish with red onion and pecans.
4. Garnish with parsley and grapefruit segments.

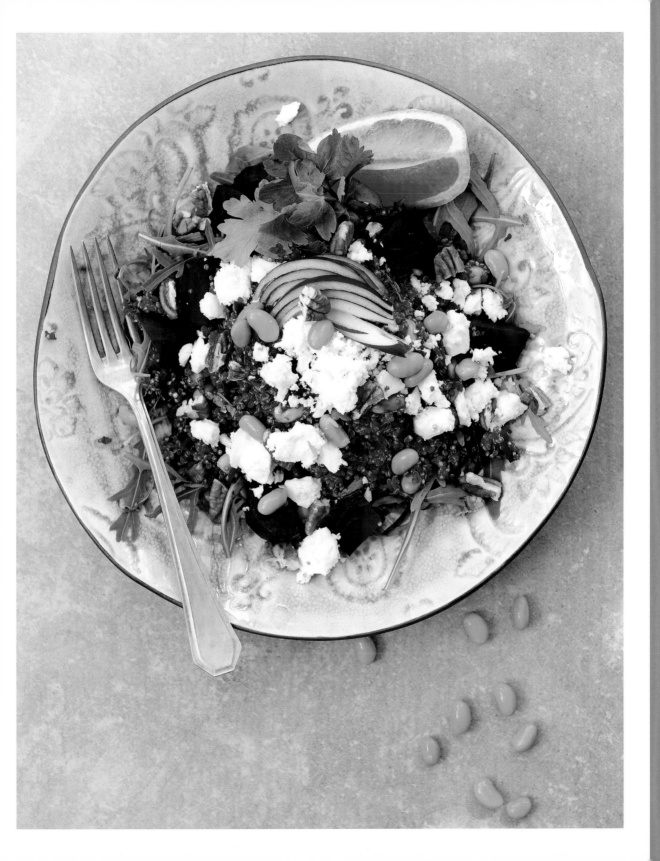

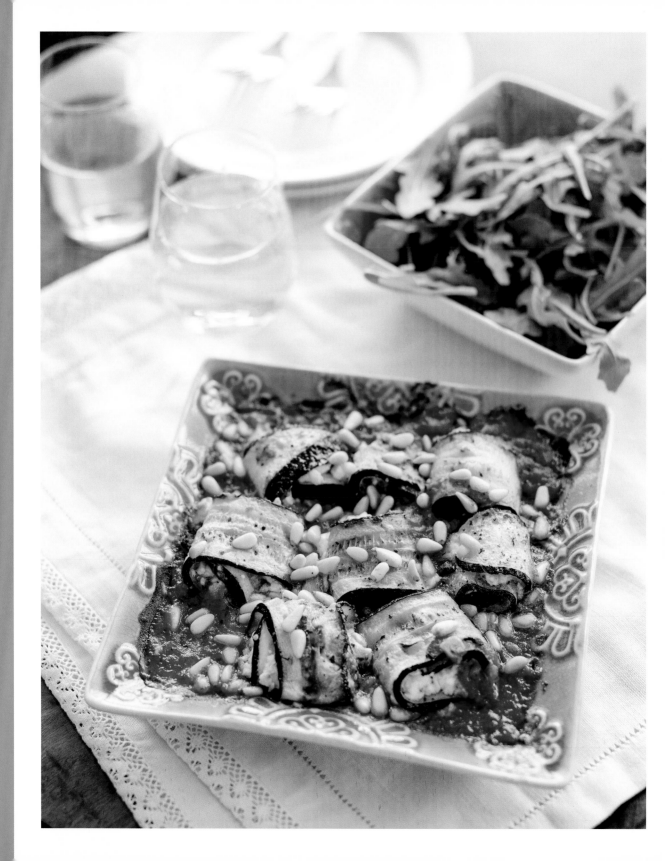

Zucchini Roll-ups
WITH FETA CHEESE

Tasty, filling, and easy to prepare zucchini roll-ups. They're also practical because they can be prepared a day in advance.

420 CALORIES/SERVES 2

1 medium zucchini
1 tablespoon olive oil
Salt
Black pepper
Dried herbs—choose your favorites
2 tablespoons green pesto (see p. 58, or use store-bought)
2¾ ounces (75 g) feta cheese
¾ ounce (20 g) pine nuts, for garnish
1¾ ounce (50 g) arugula, for garnish

Tomato sauce

½ yellow onion
1 small clove garlic
1 teaspoon olive oil
1 can (7 ounces or 200 g) crushed tomatoes
1 teaspoon Mediterranean herb mix
1 teaspoon honey
Salt
Black pepper

1. Preheat the oven to 440°F (225°C). Cut the zucchini lengthwise into slices about ¼ inch (½ cm) thick. Heat the olive oil in a skillet. Fry the zucchini slices for a minute or two on each side to soften them. Season with salt and pepper and some dried herbs. Transfer the slices to a platter.

2. Spread some pesto on each zucchini slice. Crumble the feta cheese over them and roll up the slices. Place the slices in an oiled oven-safe dish.

3. Sliver the onion and finely chop the garlic clove for the tomato sauce. Heat some oil in a saucepan. Cook the onion and garlic for a few minutes. Mix in the crushed tomatoes, the Mediterranean herb mix, and the honey. Let cook for about 5 minutes and season with salt and pepper.

4. Pour the tomato sauce over the zucchini roll-ups (you can prepare them in advance up to this point). Top with pine nuts and bake in the oven for about 15 minutes. Serve with a light arugula salad.

Greek Poke Bowl

Chickpeas, feta cheese, and ajvar pepper relish make an exciting combination! Try it also with other legume combinations.

685 CALORIES/SERVES 2

1 can (14 ounces or 400 g) chickpeas
Juice from ½ lemon
1 tablespoon olive oil
2 tablespoons chopped parsley
½ red onion, finely chopped
½ red bell pepper, finely chopped
Salt
Black pepper
2¼ ounces (65 g) mixed lettuce
5¼ ounces (150 g) feta cheese
3½ ounces (100 g) grilled bell peppers—from a jar
6 cherry tomatoes
6 black olives
Sprigs of parsley, for garnish
Lemon slices, for garnish
Slivers of red onion, optional
3⅓ fluid ounces (1 dl) ajvar relish

1. Rinse the chickpeas in cold water. Drain them well and put them in a bowl. Mix in lemon juice, olive oil, parsley, red onion, and bell pepper, and season with salt and black pepper.
2. Cover the bottom of two deep bowls with lettuce leaves, and place the chickpea salad on top. Crumble the feta cheese on top and place this and the grilled red pepper in the bowl next to the salad.
3. Cut the tomatoes into pieces and place them and the olives along the bowl's edge. Garnish with parsley, lemon slices, and the optional red onion slivers. Serve with ajvar relish.

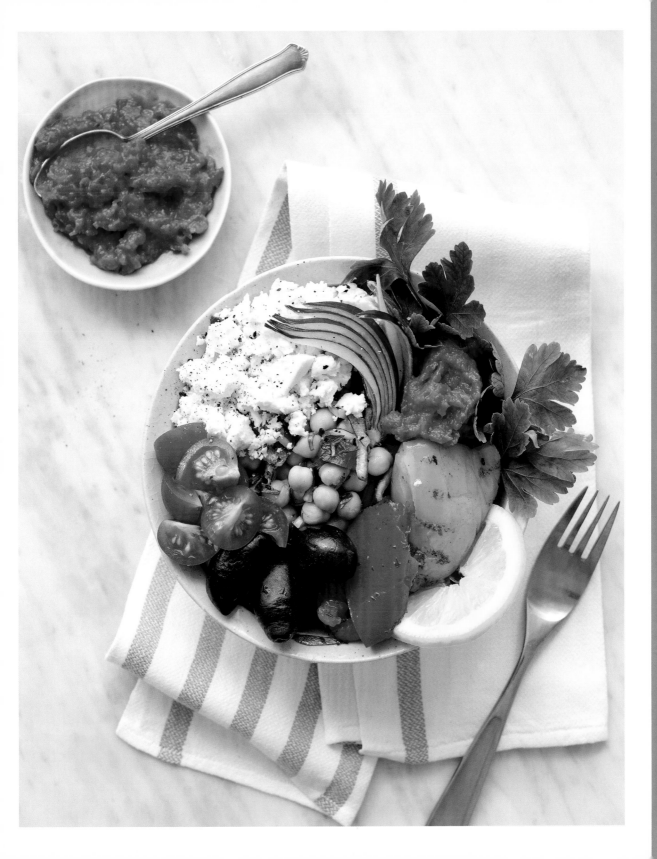

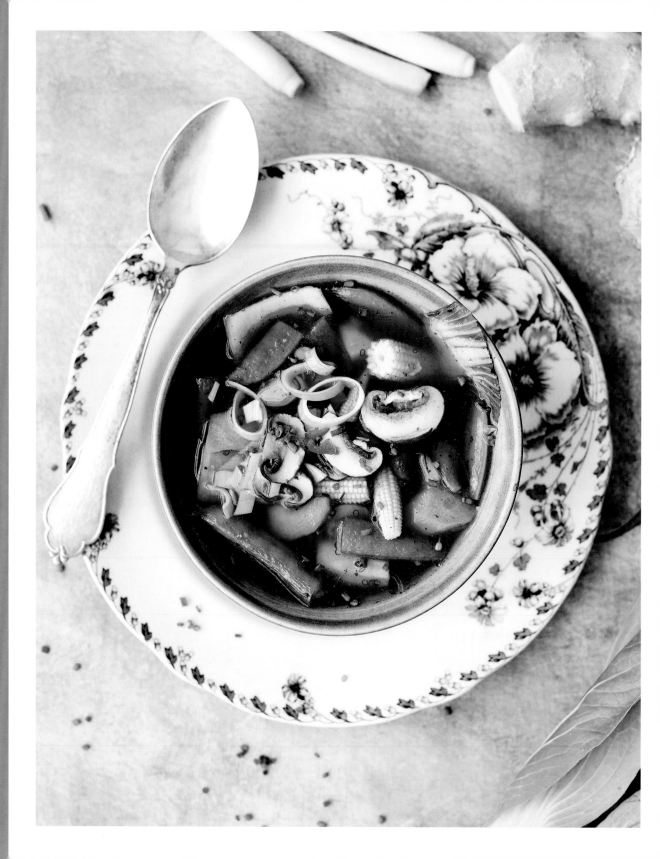

Asian Mushroom Soup

A total favorite! It can be varied in so many ways using the vegetables you already have in the refrigerator. Great both for lunch and dinner, and also works as a satisfying snack.

150 CALORIES/SERVES 2

2 cups (5 dl) water
1 chicken stock cube
1 tablespoon soy sauce
2 tablespoons mango chutney
½ red chili, chopped
1 tablespoon fresh ginger, grated
1 clove garlic, grated
7 ounces (200 g) pinewood/blushing wood mushrooms
2 inches (5 cm) leek
1 carrot
1¾ ounces (50 g) sugar snap peas
3½ ounces (100 g) baby corn
1 stalk lemongrass
Salt
Black pepper
Approximately 9 ounces (250 g) bok choy

1. In a large saucepan bring the water, stock cube, soy sauce, and mango chutney to a boil. Mix in the chopped chili, grated ginger, and garlic.
2. Slice the mushrooms and the leek. Peel and thinly slice the carrot. Open the sugar snap peas and the baby corn, and julienne the lemongrass.
3. Mix it all in the saucepan and season with salt and pepper. Let it simmer for 2 minutes. Slice the bok choy leaves and fold them into the soup just before serving.

Portobello Mushroom
WITH MOZZARELLA CHEESE

These cheese-covered mushrooms are filling and satisfying. The flavor reminds me of pizza, and it can be easily modified by using different fillings.

330 CALORIES/SERVES 2

2 large portobello mushrooms
Salt
Black pepper
4½ ounces (125 g) mozzarella cheese
3½ ounces (100 g) cherry tomatoes
2 tablespoons chopped yellow onion

Pesto

2½ ounces (70 g) pine nuts
1 bunch basil
1 clove garlic
2 teaspoons honey
Salt
Black pepper
2½ fluid ounces (¾ dl) olive oil

To serve

1 ounce (30 g) arugula

1. Preheat the oven to 400°F (200°C). Remove the mushroom stems and place the mushroom caps, outer side facing down, in a small ovenproof dish. Season them with some salt and pepper. Leave the mushrooms in the oven for about 5 minutes.
2. Place all the pesto ingredients—except the oil—in a food processor and mix to a coarse consistency. Finish by adding the oil bit by bit while the food processor is running.
3. Slice the mozzarella and cut some of the tomatoes into chunks. Divide evenly over the mushroom along with the pesto. Top with onion and season with a bit of salt and pepper.
4. Bake in the oven for about 10 minutes and serve with an arugula salad and the remaining tomatoes.

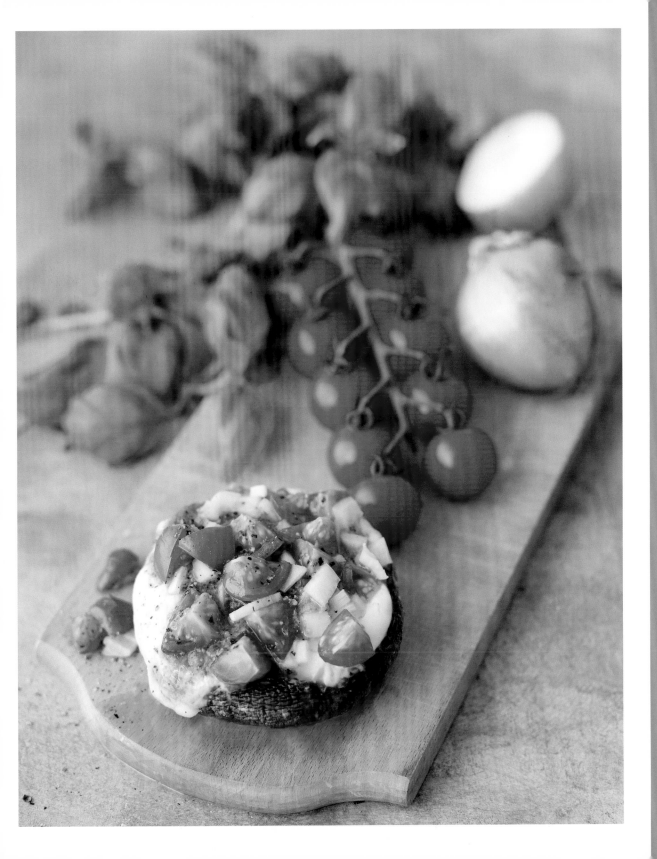

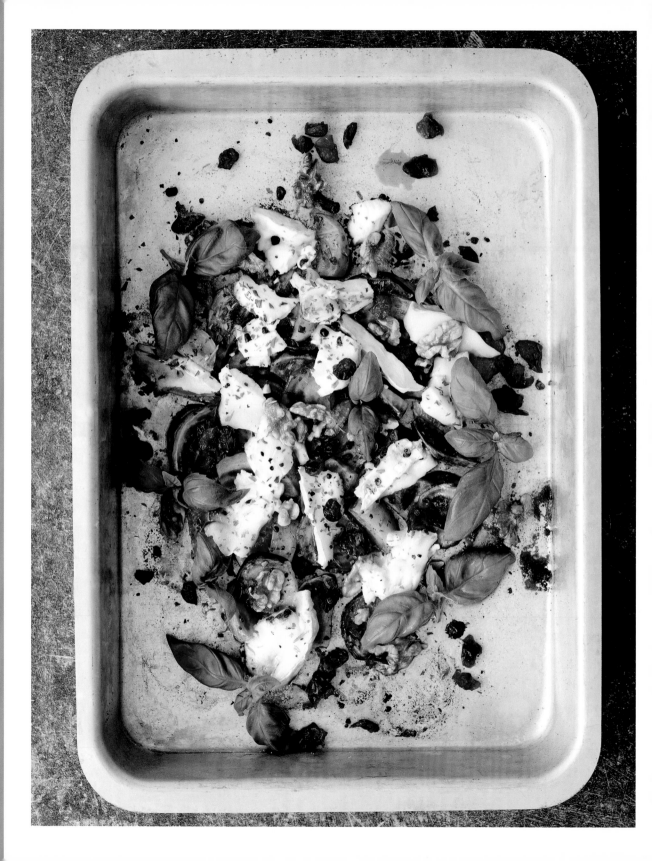

Roasted Golden Beets
WITH CHÈVRE

Food should be pleasing to both the palate and the eyes. This is much more important than people think. Here is a beautiful dish that can be modified using different root vegetables and cheeses. And, it takes care of itself in the oven.

575 CALORIES/SERVES 4

1 pound (500 g) yellow beets
1 tablespoon olive oil
1 tablespoon honey
Salt
Black pepper
⅕ teaspoon (1 krm) dried French herbs
7 ounces (200 g) chèvre
3 ½ ounces (100 g) walnuts

Topping

1¾ ounces (50 g) dried cranberries
⅕ teaspoon (1krm) dried French herbs
Fresh basil leaves

1. Preheat the oven to 425°F (220°C). Peel the beets and cut them into segments. Scatter the segments on a rimmed baking sheet and drizzle with olive oil and honey.
2. Season with salt, black pepper, and dried herbs. Crumble the chèvre over the top and sprinkle with the walnuts.
3. Bake in the oven for 15 to 20 minutes. Top with cranberries, dried herbs, and basil leaves.

CARROT FALAFEL WITH
Tomato Salad

Vegetarian chickpea burgers. Dried chickpeas make the tastiest burgers, but remember to plan in some soaking time for the chickpeas.

435 CALORIES/SERVES 4

2 cups (5 dl) dried chickpeas

3⅔ ounces (1 dl) chopped frozen parsley

2 tablespoons tahini

1 yellow onion

3 small cloves garlic

½ tablespoon olive oil + 1 tablespoon for frying

1 tablespoon organic and gluten-free stock powder

1 teaspoon cumin

Salt

Black pepper

1 tablespoon sweet chili sauce

3 carrots

Tomato salad

8¾ ounces (250 g) tomatoes, mix of colors

½ red onion

1 red chili

Leaves from a bunch of mint, divided

Juice from 1 lime

1 tablespoon olive oil

Salt

Black pepper

Seeds from ½ pomegranate, for garnish

1. Soak the chickpeas for 6 to 8 hours. Drain off the water and place the chickpeas in a food processor. Add parsley and tahini and mix quickly.

2. Chop the onion and garlic. Heat some oil in a skillet and fry the onion and garlic for a minute or two. Add the stock powder, cumin, salt, pepper, and sweet chili sauce. Pour it all into the food processor and mix to a smooth mixture.

3. Coarsely grate the carrots and add them to the mixture. Form 8 burgers and fry them in oil over medium heat for about 3 minutes on each side.

4. Make the tomato salad while the burgers are cooking. Halve the tomatoes and place them in a bowl. Thinly slice the red onion and finely chop the chili and mint—save a few mint leaves for garnish. Mix everything in a bowl along with lime juice, oil, salt, and pepper.

5. Place burgers and tomato salad on plates. Garnish with mint and pomegranate seeds

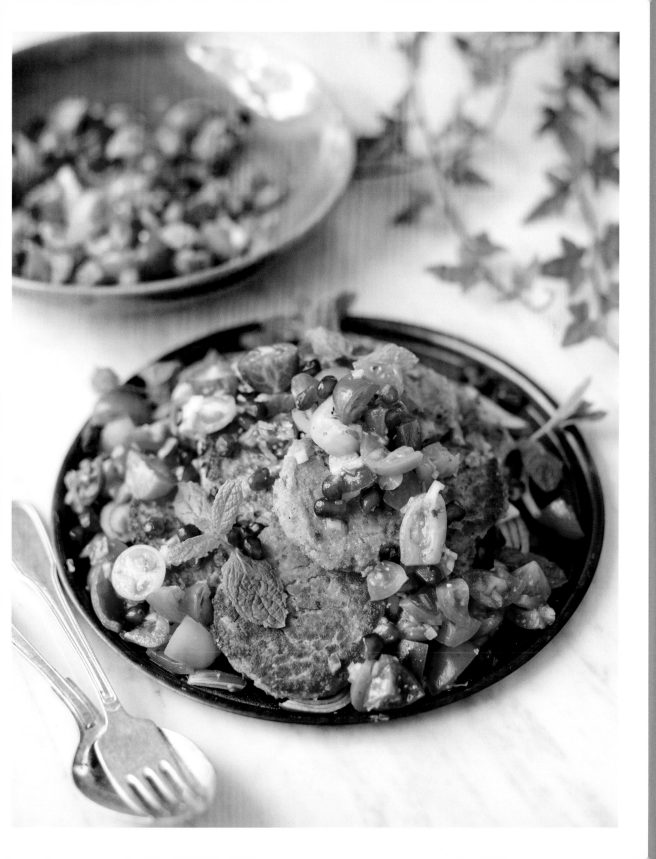

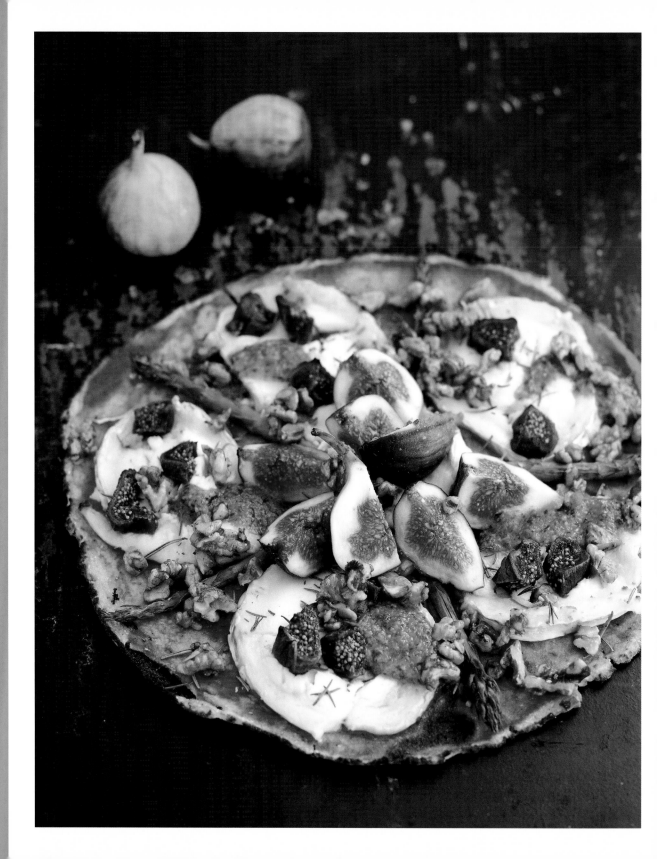

Cauliflower Pizza
WITH CHÈVRE AND FIGS

It's difficult to find a more beautiful pizza! The chèvre, fig, and asparagus flavor combination is wonderful!

797 CALORIES/SERVES 2

Pizza dough

½ medium cauliflower
4 tablespoons (¼ dl) pecorino cheese, grated
4 tablespoons (¼ dl) buffalo mozzarella, grated
1 egg
½ teaspoon salt
⅕ teaspoon (1 krm) garlic powder

Tomato sauce

½ yellow onion
1 teaspoon olive oil
1 small clove garlic, pressed
½ can crushed tomatoes, approximately 7 ounces (200 g)
⅕ teaspoon (1 krm) Mediterranean herbs
Salt
Black pepper

Topping

7 ounces (200 g) chèvre, cut in slices
1 + ½ tablespoon honey, divided
3 dried figs
5 stalks green asparagus
4 tablespoons (½ dl) chopped walnuts
3 fresh figs
4 tablespoons (½ dl) green pesto (see p. 58, or use store bought)
2 teaspoons dried rosemary

1. Preheat the oven to 400°F (200°C). Separate the cauliflower into florets and run them in a food processor until they become crumbs. Place the cauliflower in a saucepan, cover with water, and bring to a boil. Let simmer until all cauliflower is soft, about 5 minutes. Drain the water thoroughly, place the cauliflower in a clean dish towel, and wring out the remaining water.

2. Return the cauliflower to the food processor along with the remaining ingredients for the pizza dough. Mix until dough forms. Place the dough on a baking sheet covered in parchment paper and press it out until it is even and thin. Prebake the dough for 20 minutes. Raise the heat to 475°F (250°C).

3. Finely chop the onion and fry it for a few minutes in a skillet with some oil. Add the garlic, crushed tomatoes, and spices and let simmer for a few minutes. Blend the sauce until smooth.

4. Divide the tomato sauce evenly over the pizza dough and cover with the slices of chèvre. Season with salt and black pepper and drizzle a tablespoon of honey over the cheese. Chop the dried figs and sprinkle them over the honey. Add the asparagus and bake for 12–15 minutes.

5. Roast the walnuts in a dry skillet, stirring the whole time. Finish by drizzling one-half tablespoon honey into the walnuts and stirring. Cut the fresh figs into segments and place them and the walnuts on the pizza. Dot the pizza with pesto and finish by sprinkling it with rosemary.

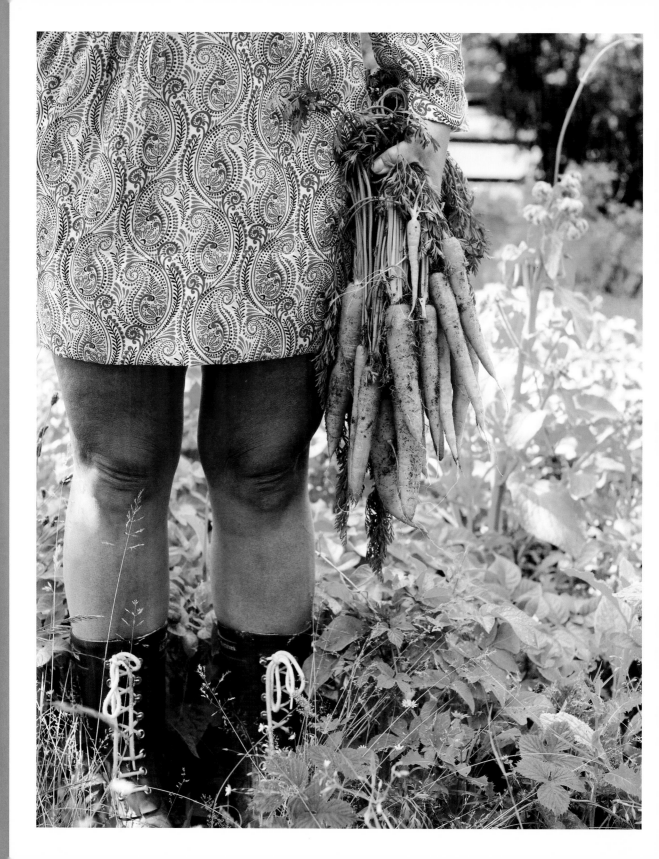

DETOX
Meal Schedule

DURATION: 2 WEEKS
WEIGHT LOSS: APPROXIMATELY 8¾ POUNDS (4 KG)

The focus here is on cleansing and cleaning up. You'll eat a vegetarian diet based on raw natural and organic ingredients, and get a real jolt of energy. Plus, you'll quickly lose some weight!

Many experience a real improvement in health after finishing this kickstart. It's for you if, for example, you have problems with low energy, gut and digestion issues, bloating, body aches and pains, and allergic reactions to pollen or outbreaks of asthma. You will lose about 8 ¾ pounds (4 kg) in two weeks, and your body measurements will change radically, because among other things, you'll lose a lot of fluid that would otherwise remain in the body's tissues.

Your caloric intake is between 425 and 2,076 calories per day. There are fasting days in the schedule when you will eat below 500 calories per day. Days of irregular caloric intake in tandem with intermittent fasting cause quick weight loss. The body never has the opportunity to get used to a certain amount of calories, and will therefore kick your metabolism into higher gear.

You'll eat plenty of vegetables, some fruit and berries, plain nuts and seeds, some root vegetables and gluten-free quinoa, and goat and sheep cheeses.

It's better if you can avoid drinking coffee and black tea during the detox, but it isn't a must. Maybe you can try to decrease your consumption and only drink a cup a day?

To avoid chaining you to the stove for the duration of the detox, I've designed the schedule so yesterday's dinner will occasionally become today's lunch or dinner. You can swap recipes between lunch and dinner the same day, but you can't switch them around between days. The dishes are not suitable for freezing and should be eaten within three days.

If you enjoy the slightly spicy Detox My Morning beverage (see p. 150) drink it every morning if you like. It's cleansing, and great for the immune system and pH level. (Cayenne pepper boosts metabolism a bit!)

DAY	BREAKFAST	LUNCH	DINNER
Monday **516 calories**	Detox My Morning, p. 150 (75 calories)	Detox Soup, p. 41 (150 calories)	Bell Pepper in Feta Cheese Gratin, p. 46 (291 calories)
Tuesday **1,250 calories**	Chia Seed Porridge, p. 35 (269 calories)	Bell Pepper in Feta Cheese Gratin (291 calories), *leftovers*	Fruity Feta Cheese Salad in a Jar, p. 49 (690 calories)
Wednesday **425 calories**	Detox My Morning, p. 150 (75 calories)	Rice wraps with mango and curry sauce, p. 42 (200 calories)	Detox Soup (150 calories), *leftovers*
Thursday **937 calories**	¼ cup (1 dl) soy yogurt (42 calories) with ⅓ cup (¾ dl) Quinoa Granola, p. 36 (175 calories)	Rice Wraps with Mango and Curry Sauce (200 calories), *leftovers*	Beet Quinoa with Feta Cheese, p. 50 (520 calories)
Friday **1,307 calories**	1 pitcher Green Energy Drink, p. 154 (367 calories)	Beet Quinoa with Feta Cheese (520 calories), *leftovers*	Zucchini Roll-ups with Feta Cheese, p. 53 (420 calories)
Saturday **2,076 calories**	Yellow Sunshine Smoothie, p. 153 (481 calories)	Zucchini Roll-ups with Feta Cheese (420 calories), *leftovers*	Greek Poke Bowl, p. 54 (685 calories) Berry Sorbet, p. 184 (75 calories) Brie Gratin with Pecans, p. 194 (415 calories)
Sunday **910 calories**	Detox My Morning, p. 150 (75 calories)	Greek Poke Bowl (685 calories), *leftovers*	Asian Mushroom Soup, p. 57 (150 calories)

DAY	BREAKFAST	LUNCH	DINNER
Monday **555 calories**	Detox My Morning, p. 150 (75 calories)	Asian Mushroom Soup, p. 57 (150 calories)	Portobello with Mozzarella Cheese, p. 58 (330 calories)
Tuesday **1,149 calories**	Soy yogurt with citrus and pistachios, p.32 (244 calories)	Portobello with Mozzarella Cheese (330 calories), *leftovers*	Roasted Golden Beets with Chèvre, p. 61 (575 calories)
Wednesday **461 calories**	2 servings Bloody Mary Cleansing Beauty, p. 162 (145 calories)	Detox Soup, p. 41 (150 calories)	2 servings Kale Smoothie, p. 32 (166 calories)
Thursday **1,087 calories**	¼ cup (1 dl) soy yogurt (42 calories) with $\frac{1}{3}$ cup (3/4 dl) Quinoa Granola, p. 36 (175 calories)	Roasted Golden Beets with Chèvre (575 calories), *leftovers* 2 portions Bloody Mary Cleansing Beauty (145 calories), *leftovers*	Detox Soup (150 calories), *leftovers*
Friday **1,036 calories**	2 servings Kale Smoothie, p. 32 (166 calories)	Vegetables with hummus, p.44 (435 calories)	Carrot Falafel with Tomato Salad, p. 62 (435 calories)
Saturday **1,621 calories**	Sesame Seed Crackers with Pecorino Cheese, p. 38 (260 calories)	Vegetables with Hummus, p. 44 (435 calories) *or* 1 pitcher Green Energy Drink, p. 154 (367 calories)	Cauliflower Pizza with Chèvre and Figs, p. 65 (737 calories)
Sunday **1,307 calories**	Detox My Morning p.150 (75 calories)	Cauliflower Pizza with Chèvre and Figs (737 calories), *leftovers*	Carrot Falafel with Tomato Salad (435 calories), *leftovers*

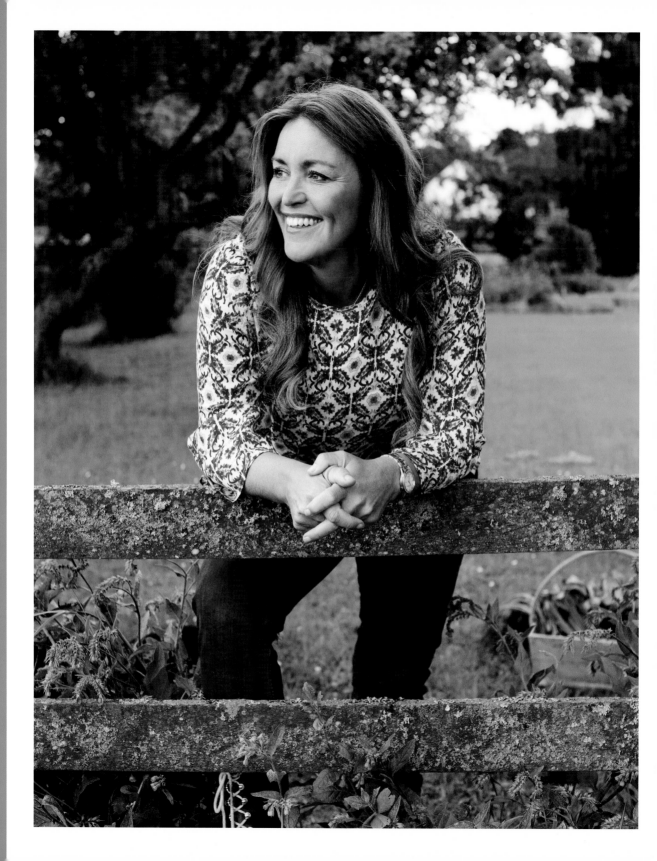

VEGETARIAN

– RECIPES AND MEAL SCHEDULE –

Many who follow vegetarian-based nutrition base their meals on carbo-hydrates, and unfortunately on refined carbohydrates. This vegetarian kickstart lasts two weeks and illustrates how you can eat a vegetarian diet and lose some weight at the same time. In addition, you'll develop a healthier and more balanced blood glucose level.

It's important to find enjoyment and inspiration when you change your dietary habits. You'll get this with my green recipes in this chapter—vegetarian options that promote good health. I have created the recipes in the schedule to contain a maximum amount of vitamins and minerals, as well as the so-important enzymes that are good for your digestion. And they are easy to prepare.

The recipes are based on a low-carbohydrate diet that is gluten-free, free of refined sugar, and to a great degree free of cow's milk. The schedule at the end of this chapter is set up so the caloric amount changes each day. There are also two intermittent fasting days during the week, when you eat only about 500 calories a day. There's also a variation where you skip breakfast and make lunch your first meal. That gives you sixteen hours of fasting and an eight-hour eating window. This is great for the metabolism!

I hope you will enjoy my colorful and easy-to-prepare recipes that are suitable for all—older, younger, and everyone in between.

Pomegranate Beverage
WITH MELON AND ALMONDS

A filling and delicious drink that will light up your morning.

426 CALORIES/SERVES 2

¼ watermelon
1 pomegranate
3⅓ ounces (1 dl) raspberries, frozen + a few extra for topping
1 small banana
3⅓ ounces (1 dl) almonds
3⅓ fluid ounces (1 dl) almond milk

1. Remove the watermelon seeds and cut away the peel. Cut the watermelon into chunks.
2. Remove the seeds from the pomegranate and put aside a few seeds for garnish. Place watermelon chunks and pomegranate seeds in a blender and add raspberries, banana, and almonds. Blend and thin with the almond milk.
3. Pour into glasses and top with raspberries and pomegranate seeds.

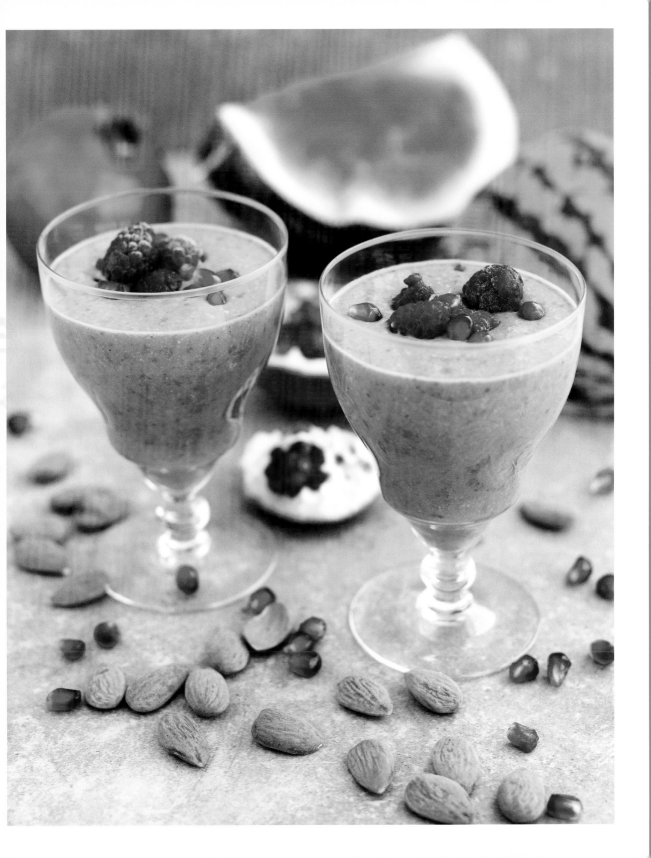

Soy Yogurt
WITH BERRIES AND MANGO

Go for a plain soy yogurt and top it with fruit and berries. Here you are free to swap out the fruits and berries for any of your own favorites.

148 CALORIES/SERVES 1

½ **mango**
3⅓ **fluid ounces (1 dl) plain soy yogurt**
1¾ **ounces (½ dl) fresh strawberries**
1¾ **ounces (½ dl) fresh raspberries**
3⅓ **ounces (1 dl) fresh blueberries**

1. Cut the mango into small pieces.
2. Pour the yogurt into a bowl and sprinkle mango and berries on top.

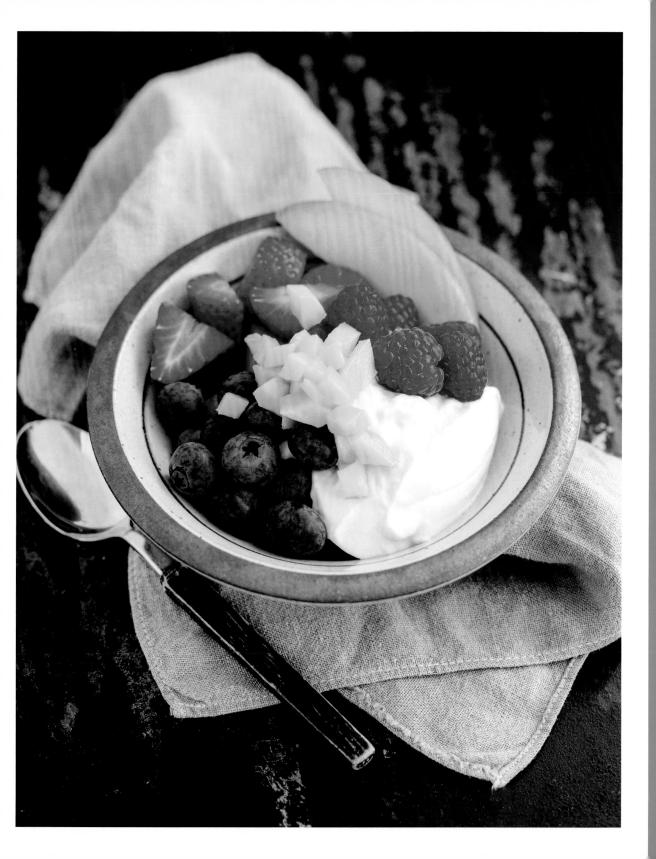

CHOCOLATE SMOOTHIE BOWL
with Chia Seeds

A breakfast bowl that's almost too good to be true—and also extremely filling!

300 CALORIES/SERVES 2

2 tablespoons chia seeds

5 fluid ounces (1½ dl) oat milk

⅕ teaspoon (1 krm) vanilla powder

1 avocado

3⅓ ounces (1 dl) diced mango, frozen

5 dried pitted dates

2 tablespoons cocoa

Topping

3⅓ fluid ounces (1 dl) lingonberries or cranberries

1 plum

2 teaspoons chia seeds

1. Mix chia seeds, oat milk, and vanilla powder in a bowl. Stir the mixture after 5 minutes.
2. Peel the avocado and remove the pit. Cut out a few slices and place the rest of the avocado in a food processor together with the mango, dates, cocoa, and the chia seed mixture.
3. Blend to a smooth mixture and pour it into a bowl.
4. Top with lingonberries, slices of plum, and avocado. Sprinkle with some chia seeds and serve.

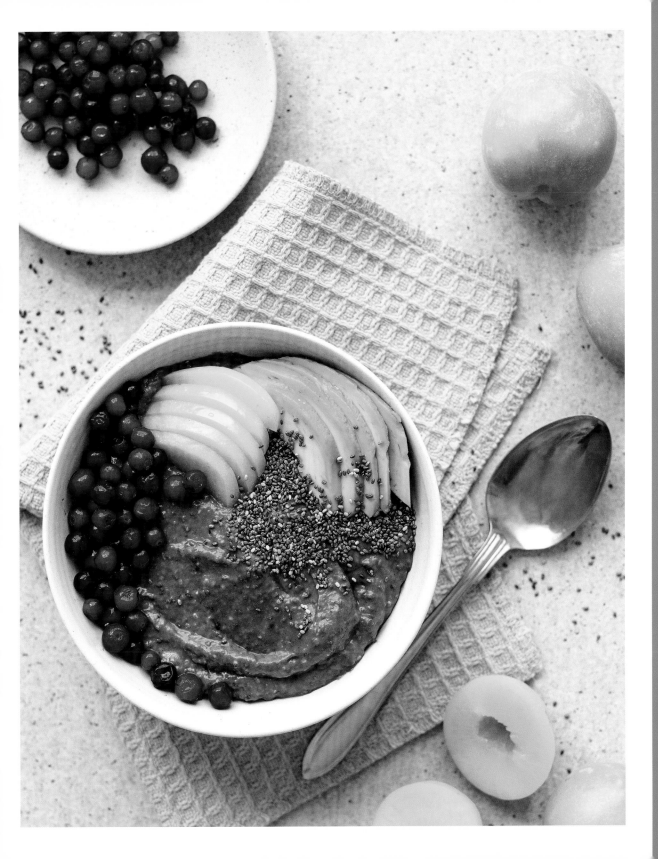

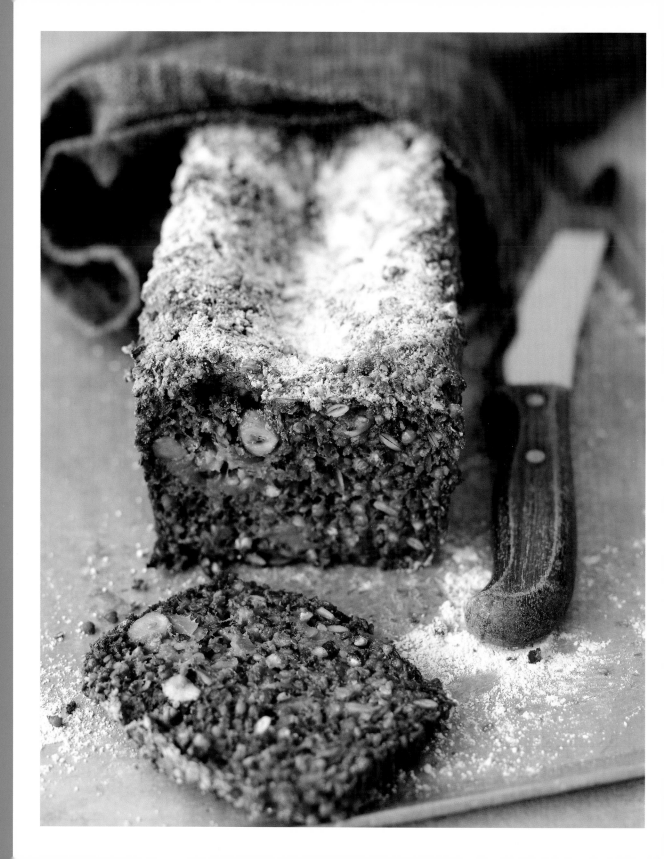

Sprouted Bread
WITH APRICOTS

An easy to bake and sturdy bread that keeps well for several days.
A loaf with wonderful flavor and texture!

192 CALORIES/MAKES 12 SLICES

- 7 ounces (200 g) sprouted buckwheat (approximately 6¾ ounces/2 dl unsprouted grain)
- 1 tablespoon fiber husk
- 3⅓ ounces (1 dl) flaxseeds
- 3⅓ ounces (1 dl) sesame seeds
- 6¾ fluid ounces (2 dl) water, boiling
- 6¾ ounces (2 dl) oat flour + more for sprinkling
- 2 teaspoons baking soda
- 1½ teaspoon salt
- 5 fluid ounces (1 ½ dl) oat yogurt
- 1¾ fluid ounce (½ dl) dark Swedish* syrup
- ⅕ teaspoon (1 krm) whole aniseed
- ⅕ teaspoon (1 krm) whole fennel seed
- ⅕ teaspoon (1 krm) whole caraway seed
- 5 dried apricots
- 3⅓ ounces (1 dl) roasted pumpkin seed
- 3⅓ ounces (1 dl) roasted hazelnuts (filberts)
- Oil for the baking tin

1. Rinse the buckwheat in boiling water and then let it soak in water for about 8 hours. Drain the buckwheat in a sieve and rinse thoroughly with water. Let drain.

2. Preheat the oven to 400°F (200°C). Mix fiber husk, flaxseeds, and sesame seeds in a large bowl. Add the boiling water and let it swell for about 10 minutes. Add the sprouted buckwheat, oat flour, baking soda, salt, yogurt, Swedish syrup, and spices. Use an electric hand mixer and mix for several minutes.

3. Chop the apricots and stir them into batter along with the pumpkin seeds and nuts. Spread the batter evenly in an oiled baking pan (approximately 2 quarts). Sprinkle some oat flour on top and let it sit under a baking cloth for about 30 minutes.

4. Bake in the lower part of the oven for about 1 hour. Let the bread sit for at least 30 minutes in the pan and then turn it out onto a cooling rack. Let cool under a baking cloth.

Tip!
Bake a double batch if you have the opportunity to do so, and freeze one loaf. You can always slice it before freezing.

*Swedish syrup differs in taste from high-fructose corn syrup and can be found on Amazon.

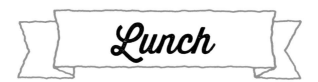
Marinated Chioggia Beets
WITH FETA CHEESE

A beautiful and colorful dish with lots of flavor!

561 CALORIES/SERVES 2

Marinade

1 tablespoon olive oil
1 tablespoon cider vinegar
1 tablespoon honey
Salt
Black pepper

4 Chioggia beets
2 carrots
1 bunch fresh chervil
5¼ ounces (150 g) feta cheese
1¾ ounces (½ dl) slivered almonds, roasted
Lemon wedges, for garnish

1. Start by making the marinade and whisk together all the ingredients in a bowl.
2. Thinly slice the Chioggia beets and carrots with a knife or a mandoline, and mix into the marinade. Marinate for 30 minutes.
3. Place the root vegetables on a platter and arrange chervil all around. Slice the feta cheese and place the slices on top. Top with almond slivers and garnish with some lemon wedges.

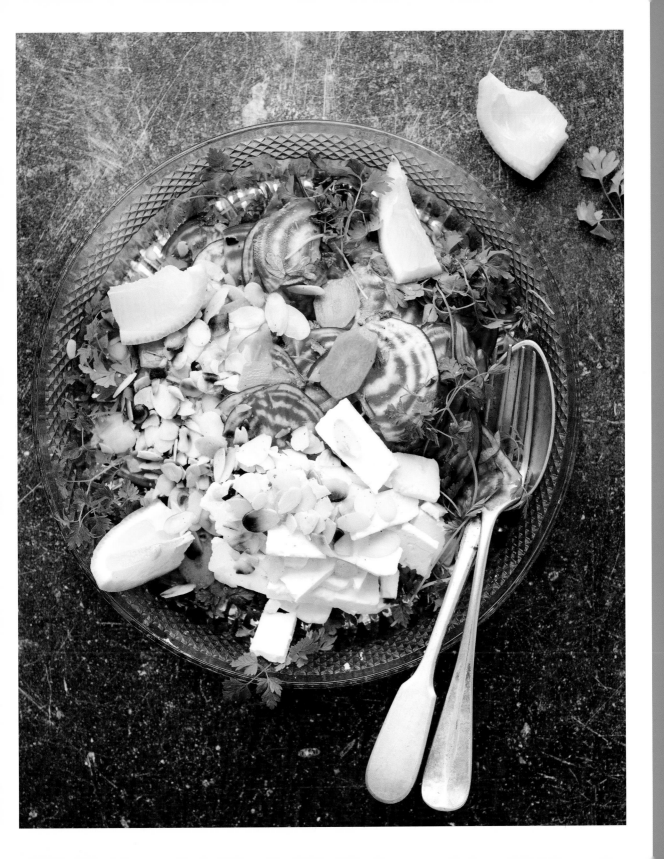

Carrot Soup
WITH GINGER

You'll pack a lot of color and flavor in this easy-to-prepare soup.

150 CALORIES/SERVES 2

1 yellow onion
2 cloves garlic
1 tablespoon olive oil
3⅓ cups (8 dl) water
1 tablespoon honey
1 pound, 1¾ ounce
  (500 g) carrots
1 tablespoon organic,
  gluten-free stock powder
2 tablespoons fresh ginger,
  grated
1 pinch chili flakes or some
  freshly chopped red chili
Salt
Black pepper

Topping

Olive oil
1 teaspoon dried herbs like
  chervil, or fresh herbs
Approximately ¼ cup
  (½ dl) Root Vegetable
  Chips (see page 198)

1. Chop the onion and garlic. Heat the olive oil in a saucepan and fry the onion and garlic for about a minute. Add the water and honey.
2. Peel and slice the carrots. Stir in carrots, stock powder, ginger, and chili in the saucepan. Let boil for 10 minutes.
3. Blend the soup until smooth and thin it with more water if necessary. Season with salt and pepper.
4. Pour the soup into bowls and drizzle with some olive oil. Sprinkle with dried or fresh herbs and top with Root Vegetable Chips.

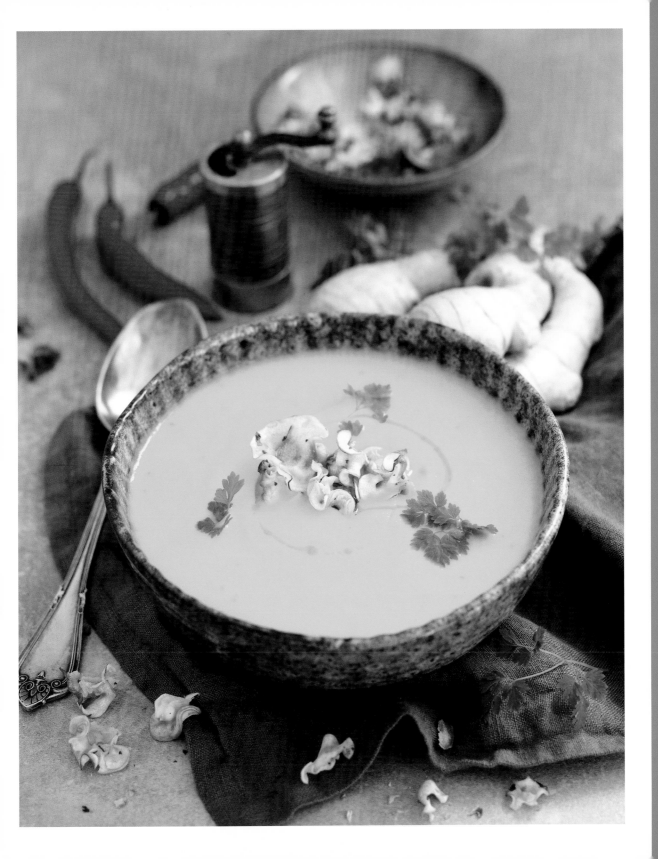

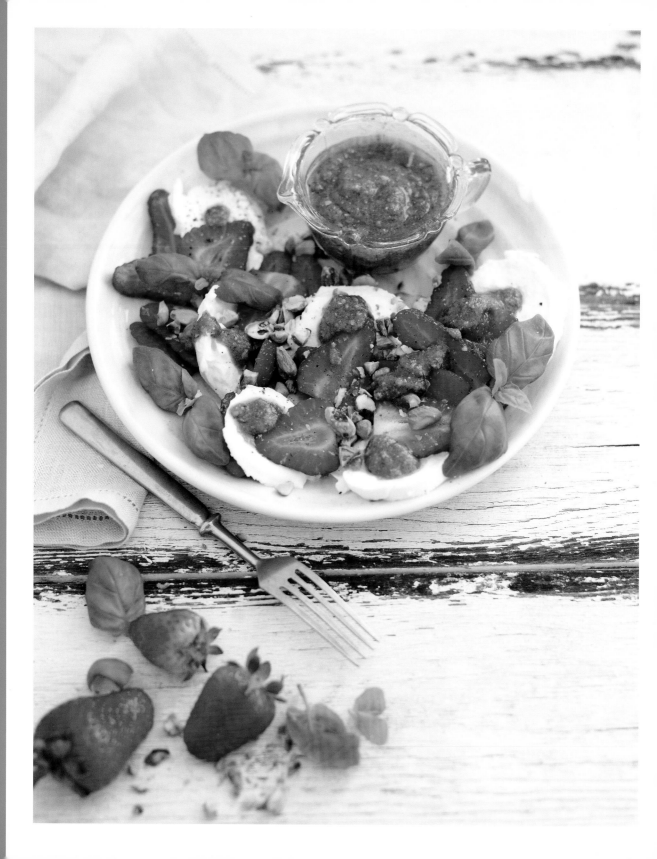

Strawberries
WITH BUFFALO MOZZARELLA AND PISTACHIO PESTO

Strawberries, mozzarella, basil, and pistachio pesto . . . what a wonderful flavor quartet!

750 CALORIES/SERVES 2

Pistachio pesto

2½ ounces (70 g) pistachios, without shells
1 bunch basil
1 clove garlic
3⅓ ounces (1 dl) pecorino cheese, grated
2 teaspoons honey
Salt
Black pepper
2½ fluid ounces (¾ dl) olive oil

Strawberries with Buffalo Mozzarella

8¾ ounces (250 g) fresh strawberries
8¾ ounces (250 g) buffalo mozzarella
Salt
Black pepper
2 tablespoons chopped pistachios
A few sprigs of basil

1. Start by making the pesto. Put all the ingredients—except the oil—in a food processor and chop coarsely. Finish by adding in the oil, bit by bit, while the food processor is running.
2. Rinse, clean, and slice the strawberries. Slice the mozzarella.
3. Divide everything between the plates and drizzle with the pesto. Season with some salt and pepper. Top with pistachios and basil.

Halloumi Burgers
WITH AJVAR PEPPER RELISH

*The ready-to-use halloumi burgers in the grocery store's frozen section are incredibly tasty.
You can also cut halloumi into slices and fry them.*

450 CALORIES/SERVES 1

1 large lettuce or cabbage leaf
½ yellow onion
1 cherry tomato
1 teaspoon olive oil
2 halloumi burgers—approximately 3⅓ ounces (100 g) each
2 slices bell pepper
3 black olives
1 tablespoon ajvar relish
1 sprig parsley, for garnish
Lemon slices, for garnish

1. Place a lettuce leaf on a plate. Slice the onion and tomato. Heat some olive oil in a skillet and fry the onion quickly, then set aside.
2. Then fry the halloumi burgers until they are nicely colored on both sides.
3. Layer bell pepper and halloumi burgers in the lettuce leaf. Top with onion, tomato, and olives. Place a dab of ajvar relish on top and garnish with parsley and lemon.

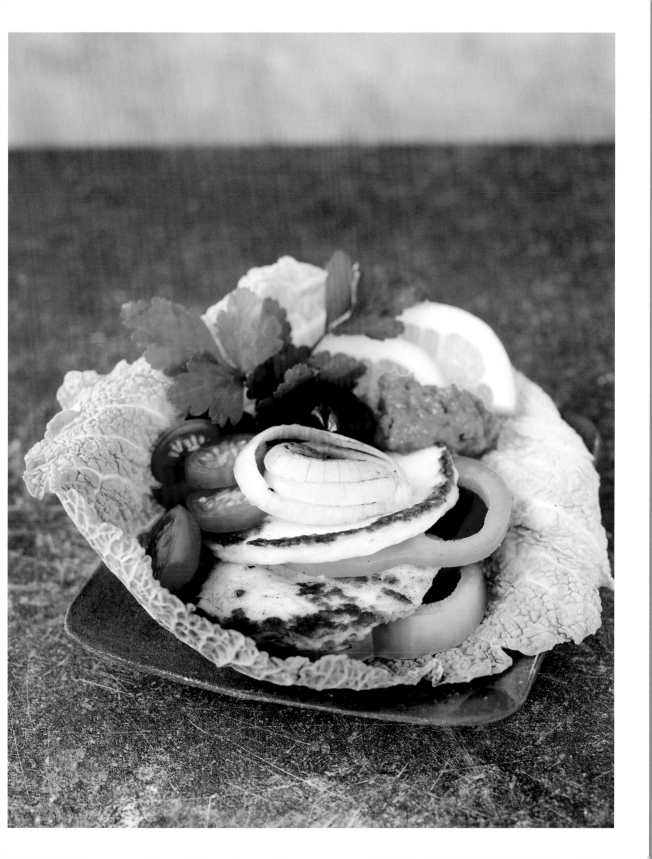

Sprouted Buckwheat Salad

WITH AJVAR PEPPER RELISH AND FETA CHEESE

When you soak buckwheat, it will release life-promoting enzymes becuase it thinks that it is preparing to sprout and grow. This makes the proteins, vitamins, and minerals more easily available to the body, and also makes them more digestible and less likely to cause flatulence.

344 CALORIES/SERVES 4

6¾ ounces (2 dl) whole buckwheat
½ red onion
1 small clove garlic
½ red bell pepper
½ yellow bell pepper
½ tablespoon olive oil
3⅓ fluid ounces (1 dl) ajvar relish
1¾ ounces (½ dl) Italian parsley, chopped
Salt
Black pepper

For serving

3½ ounces (100 g) cherry tomatoes
Fresh parsley
2¼ ounces (65 g) baby spinach

5¼ ounces (150 g) feta cheese dice in oil, drained
3⅓ ounces (1 dl) pistachios

1. Rinse the buckwheat with boiling water. Let it soak in cold water for about 8 hours. Drain the buckwheat in a sieve and rinse it thoroughly with water. Let drain.
2. Finely chop the red onion and the garlic. Cut the bell peppers into small pieces. Heat oil in a skillet and fry the vegetables. Stir in the buckwheat, ajvar relish, and parsley. Season with salt and pepper.
3. Halve the tomatoes. Cover the bottom of the plates with parsley and spinach. Divide the lukewarm buckwheat mixture on top and finish by topping it with tomatoes, feta cheese, and pistachios.

Rinsing information for buckwheat

Buckwheat contains a red substance called fagopyrin, which can irritate the eye's mucous membrane. The substance disappears when the buckwheat is rinsed, soaked, and then rinsed again.

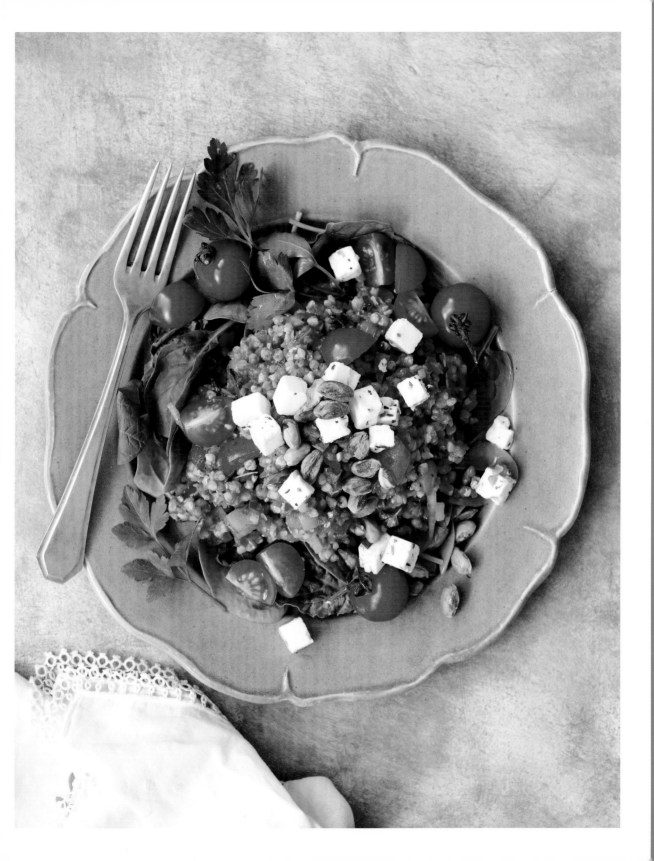

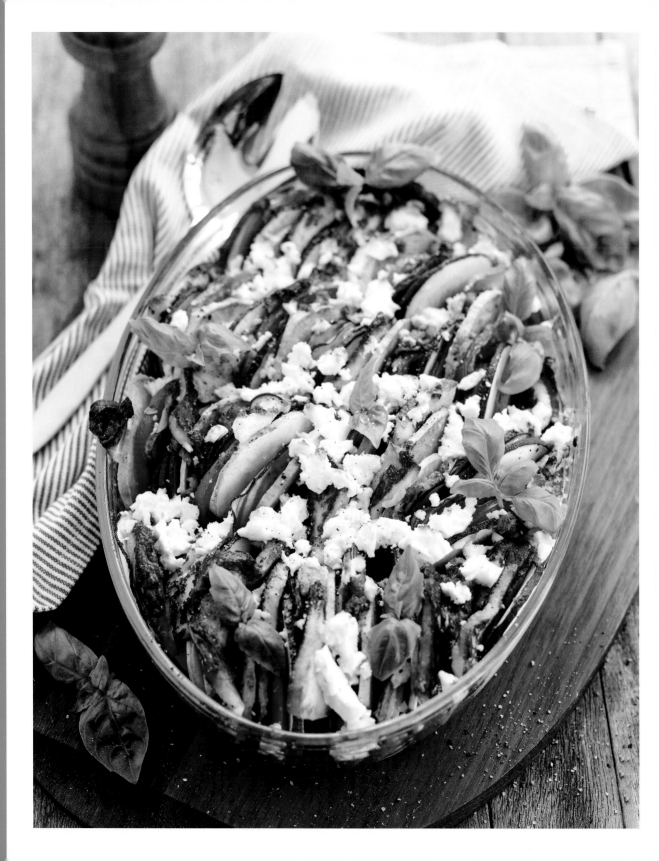

Sliced Vegetables
IN A PESTO GRATIN

An attractive and substantial dish to serve at the dinner table.
An excellent dish for brown bagging!

370 CALORIES/SERVES 4

½ sweet potato
1 parsnip
1 carrot
2 Chioggia beets or 1
  golden beet
1 zucchini
2 tomatoes
7 ounces (200 gr)
  halloumi
1 teaspoon olive oil +
  for the ovenproof dish
1¾ fluid ounce (½ dl)
  green pesto (see p. 58,
  or use store bought)
Salt
Black pepper
1 teaspoon dried basil
6¾ fluid ounces (2 dl)
  vegetable stock
5¼ ounces (150 gr) feta
  cheese
Basil leaves, for
  garnish
Leaf lettuce, for
  serving

1. Preheat the oven to 400°F (200°C). Rinse the root vegetables thoroughly, but don't peel them. Thinly slice the root vegetables, as well as the zucchini and tomatoes.
2. Slice the halloumi and fry the slices in oil until golden brown on each side. Let cool.
3. Oil an ovenproof dish, layer with standing slices of root vegetables, cheese, zucchini, and tomatoes. Dot the pesto between the slices and season with salt, pepper, and basil.
4. Drizzle with the vegetable stock and let the vegetables bake in the oven for about 20 minutes.
5. Sprinkle with crumbled feta cheese and broil for another 10 minutes. Garnish with basil leaves. Serve with a green salad.

Lentil Salad
WITH HALLOUMI AND CARROT BURGERS

Very tasty vegetarian burgers perfectly accompanied by a flavorful lentil salad.

731 CALORIES/SERVES 2

Lentil salad

3½ ounces (100 g) dried Puy lentils (small French lentils)

3½ ounces (100 g) fresh cherry tomatoes

½ bunch of fresh basil + some for garnish

½ red onion

1¾ ounce (50 g) sun-dried tomatoes in oil (preferably cherry tomatoes)

½ tablespoon olive oil

Salt

Black pepper

10 black or green olives

Halloumi and Carrot Burgers

4½ ounces (125 g) coarsely grated carrots

3½ ounces(100 g) coarsely grated halloumi

1 egg

1 pinch chili flakes

Salt flakes

1¾ fluid ounces (½ dl) sesame seed + more for breading

½ tablespoon olive oil

1. Cook the lentils in lightly salted water for about 30 minutes. Drain the water and place the lentils in a bowl.
2. Cut the fresh tomatoes into quarters. Chop the basil and red onion, and mix everything in the bowl along with sun-dried tomatoes, oil, salt, and pepper. Top with olives.
3. Mix all the ingredients for the burgers in a bowl. Shape the burgers and bread them with sesame seeds. Heat some oil in a skillet and fry the burgers for a few minutes on each side.
4. Serve the burgers with the lentil salad and garnish with basil.

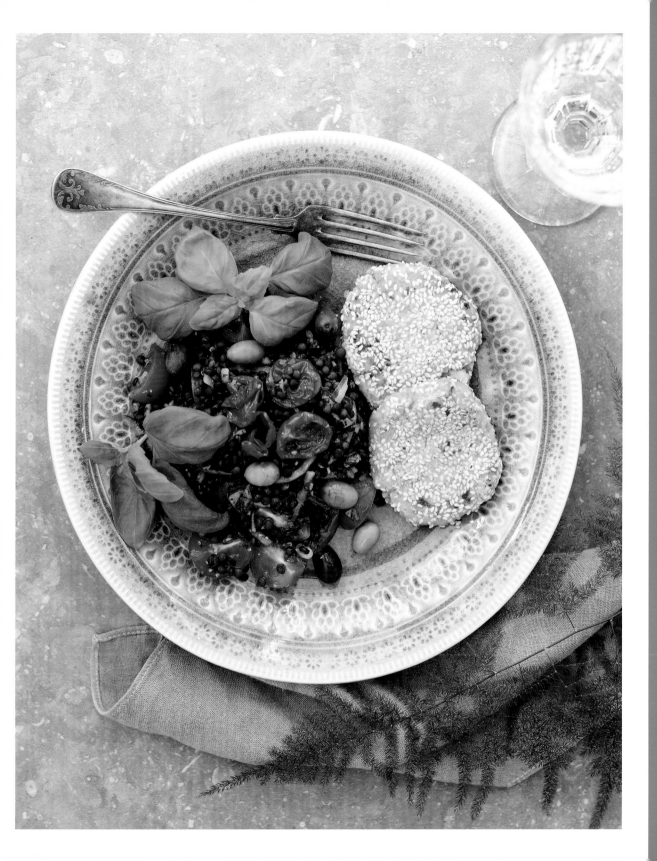

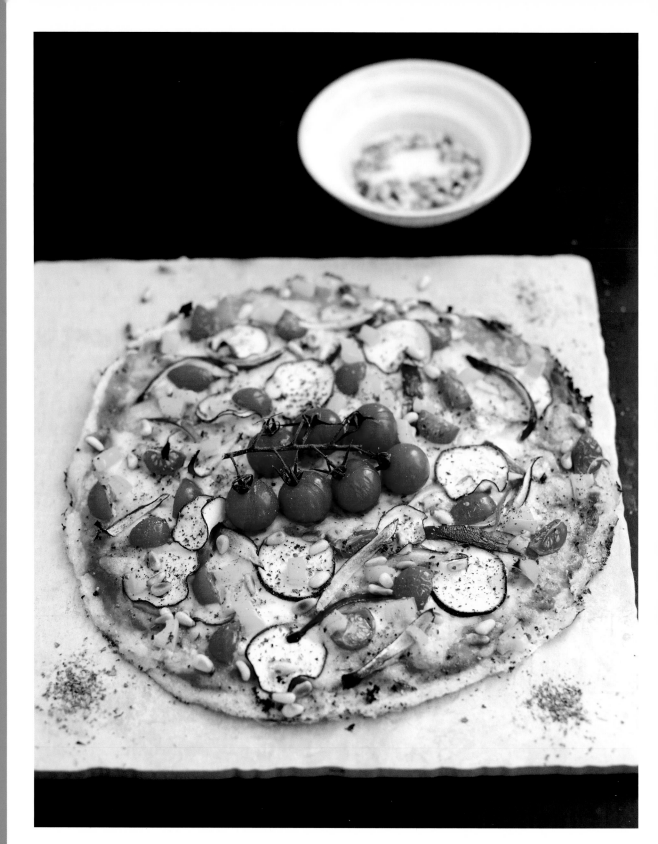

Italian
CAULIFLOWER PIZZA

An absolutely fantastic pizza that's gluten free!

389 CALORIES/SERVES 2

Pizza dough

½ **medium cauliflower**
1 ¾ **tablespoon (¼ dl) pecorino cheese, grated**
1¾ **tablespoons (¼ dl) grated buffalo mozzarella**
1 **egg**
½ **tsp salt**
⅓ **tsp (1 krm) garlic powder**

Tomato sauce

½ **yellow onion**
1 **teaspoon olive oil**
1 **small clove garlic, pressed**
½ **can crushed tomatoes— approximately 7 ounces (200 g)**
⅓ **teaspoon (1 krm) pizza spice**
Salt
Black pepper

Topping

4½ **ounces (125 g) buffalo mozzarella**
12 **cherry tomatoes**
¼ **red onion**
¾ **inch (2 cm) zucchini**
¼ **yellow bell pepper**
1 **tablespoon pine nuts**
Arugula, optional

1. Preheat the oven to 400°F (200°C). Divide the cauliflower into florets and mix them into crumbs in a food processor. Place the cauliflower crumbs in a saucepan, cover with water and let come to a boil. Let simmer until the cauliflower is soft, about 5 minutes. Drain off the water; place the cauliflower in a clean dishtowel and squeeze out the rest of the water.

2. Return the cauliflower to the food processor along with the rest of the pizza dough ingredients. Mix to form dough. Place the dough on a baking sheet lined with parchment paper and press it into a thin and even pizza base. Prebake the dough for about 20 minutes. Increase the temperature to 475°F (250°C).

3. Finely chop the onion and fry it for a few minutes in some oil in a hot skillet. Add garlic, crushed tomatoes, and spices and let it simmer for a few minutes. Blend the sauce until smooth.

4. Spread the sauce evenly over the pizza base and sprinkle with crumbled buffalo mozzarella. Cut the tomatoes into segments (perhaps save a few whole ones) and thinly slice the red onion and zucchini. Spread the vegetables over the pizza. Chop the bell pepper and sprinkle over the pizza along with the pine nuts. Season with a bit of pizza spice.

5. Bake the pizza for 15 minutes. If desired, scatter some arugula on top when ready to serve.

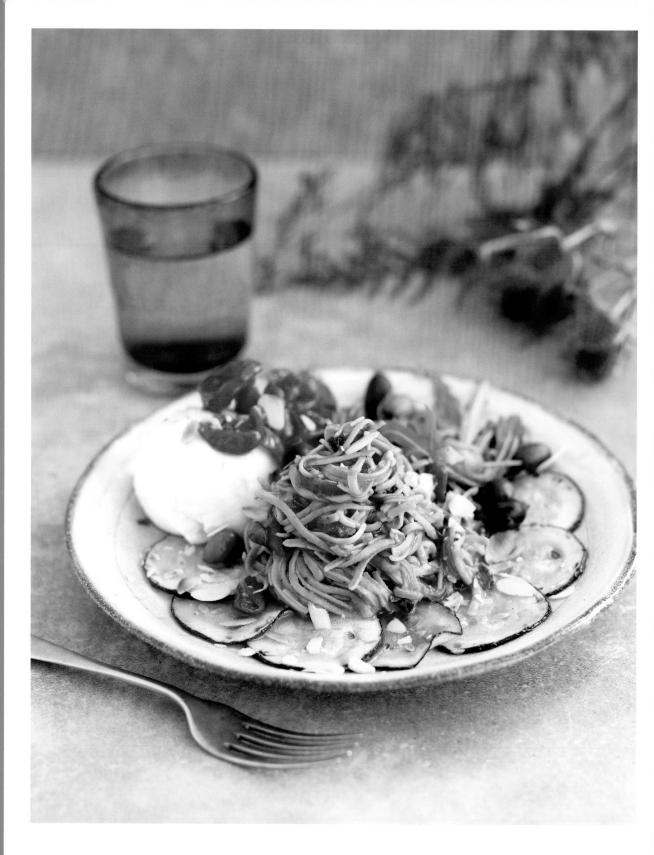

Spaghetti Pomodoro
WITH BUFFALO MOZZARELLA

Select gluten-free pasta made with beans, lentils, or soy.
There are many good varieties out there to choose from.

850 CALORIES/SERVES 2

Tomato sauce

½ yellow onion
1 small clove garlic
1 teaspoon olive oil
½ can crushed cherry tomatoes—
  approximately 7 ounces (200 g)
½ teaspoon honey
Salt
Black pepper
½ teaspoon dried herbs, such as basil and
  oregano

Spaghetti

7 ounces (200 g) bean spaghetti
1¾ ounces (½ dl) pecorino cheese, grated
½ zucchini
1 teaspoon olive oil
Salt
Black pepper
1 tablespoon dried herbs
1 ounce (30 gr) arugula
8¾ ounces (250 g) buffalo mozzarella
1 ounce (30 g) sun-dried tomatoes in oil
  (preferably cherry tomatoes)
1¾ ounces (½ dl) small olives with pits
2 tablespoons roasted slivered almonds for
  topping

1. Start by making the tomato sauce. Finely
   chop the onion and garlic. Heat some oil in a
   saucepan and fry the onion and garlic. Add
   the crushed tomatoes, honey, salt, pepper, and
   herbs. Let cook uncovered for about 10 minutes.
2. Prepare the bean spaghetti according to the
   instructions on the package. Drain off the water
   and mix in the spaghetti with the tomato sauce
   along with the grated pecorino cheese. Season
   with salt, pepper, and herbs.
3. Thinly slice the zucchini and fry the slices in
   oil for a few minutes. Season with salt, pepper,
   and herbs. Divide the zucchini between the
   plates and place arugula, mozzarella, sun-dried
   tomatoes, and olives on top.
4. Place the spaghetti mixture on top and garnish
   with slivered almonds.

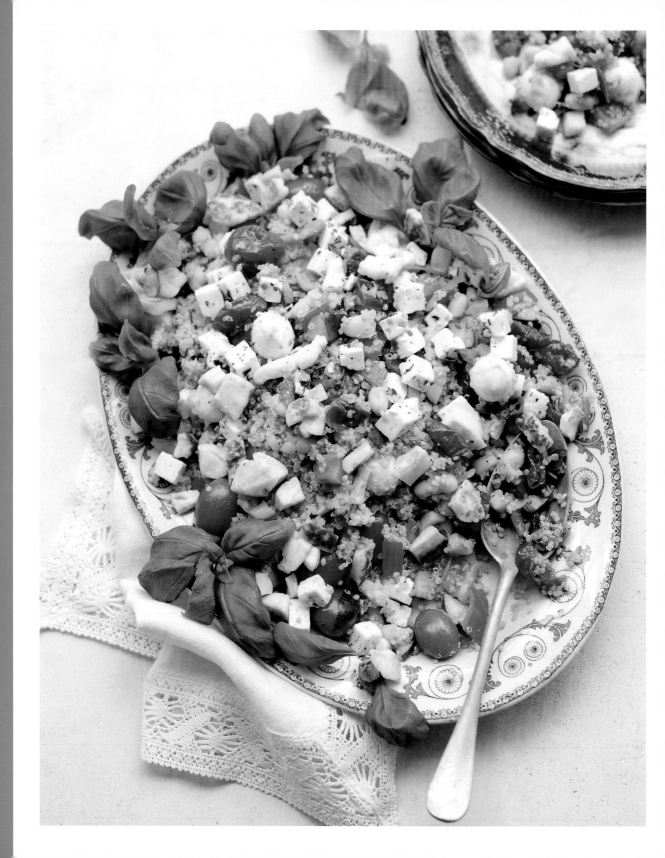

Quinoa Salad
WITH THREE CHEESES

Quinoa in the best of company—a trio of cheeses and sun-dried tomatoes.

820 CALORIES/SERVES 4

- 6¾ ounces (2 dl) quinoa
- 1 can (14 ounces or 400 g) white beans
- 3½ ounces (100 g) sun-dried tomatoes in oil (preferably cherry tomatoes)
- 3½ ounces (100 g) cherry tomatoes
- Salt
- Black pepper
- ½ red onion
- ½ zucchini
- 1 red bell pepper
- 5¼ ounces (150 g) halloumi
- 1 teaspoon olive oil
- 4½ ounces (125 g) mini mozzarella
- 4½ ounces (125 g) feta cheese dice in oil, drained
- ½ bunch fresh basil

1. Cook the quinoa according to the instructions on the package, about 13 minutes. Drain the water and place the quinoa in a bowl. Rinse the white beans in cold water and put them in the bowl together with the sun-dried tomatoes, cherry tomatoes, salt, and pepper.

2. Chop the red onion. Cut the zucchini, bell pepper, and halloumi into smaller pieces. Heat some oil in a skillet and fry everything until the halloumi has developed a nice color. Stir the mixture into the bowl and add the mozzarella and feta cheeses.

3. Chop half of the basil and mix it into the salad. Place the remaining basil along the edge of a serving platter and put the quinoa salad on the platter.

Sesame Seed–Coated Turnip Skewers
WITH NOODLE SALAD

Kelp (seaweed) noodles are extremely easy to prepare and contain almost no calories or carbohydrates. Here they are included in a salad and they pair so well with the turnip and the peanut sauce.

950 CALORIES/SERVES 2

Peanut sauce

3½ ounces (100 g) unsweetened peanut butter

2 tablespoons soy sauce

1¾ fluid ounce (½ dl) water

3½ ounce (100 g) = 3 ⅓ fluid ounces (1 dl) coconut cream

Salt

Black pepper

Turnip Skewers

10½ ounces (300 g) turnip

1 egg

1¾ fluid ounce (½ dl) sesame seeds

Salt

Black pepper

Wooden skewers

1 tablespoon olive oil

3½ ounces (100 g) fresh sugar snap peas, for serving

Noodle salad

10½ ounces (300 g) kelp/seaweed noodles

1 small clove garlic

1 teaspoon sesame oil

2 tablespoons sesame seeds + extra for sprinkling over the salad

½ tablespoon fresh grated ginger

1 tablespoon sweet chili sauce

1 tablespoon soy sauce

3½ ounces (100 g) frozen soybeans

Garnish

Fresh mint

Lime slices

Sesame seeds

1. Start by making the peanut sauce. Mix all the ingredients for the sauce in a saucepan and heat while whisking until the sauce is smooth.

2. Peel and cut the turnip into ¾-inch dice. Cook the dice in water until they are soft, about 10 minutes. Pour off the water and let the turnip cool.

3. In a deep dish, whisk the egg lightly. Mix sesame seeds, salt, and black pepper in another deep dish. Turn the turnip dice into the egg mixture and then in the plate with sesame seeds and spices. Thread the skewers with the breaded dice.

4. Heat some oil in a skillet and brown the skewers all around until they are golden.

5. Rinse the kelp/seaweed noodles in cold water. Peel and finely chop the garlic. Heat the sesame oil in a skillet and fry the garlic, sesame seeds, ginger, sweet chili sauce, and soy sauce for a minute while stirring. Stir in the kelp noodles and soybeans. Season with salt and pepper.

5. Julienne the sugar snap peas and put on the plates. Add noodle salad and skewers. Garnish with some sesame seeds, fresh mint, and lime. Serve with the peanut sauce.

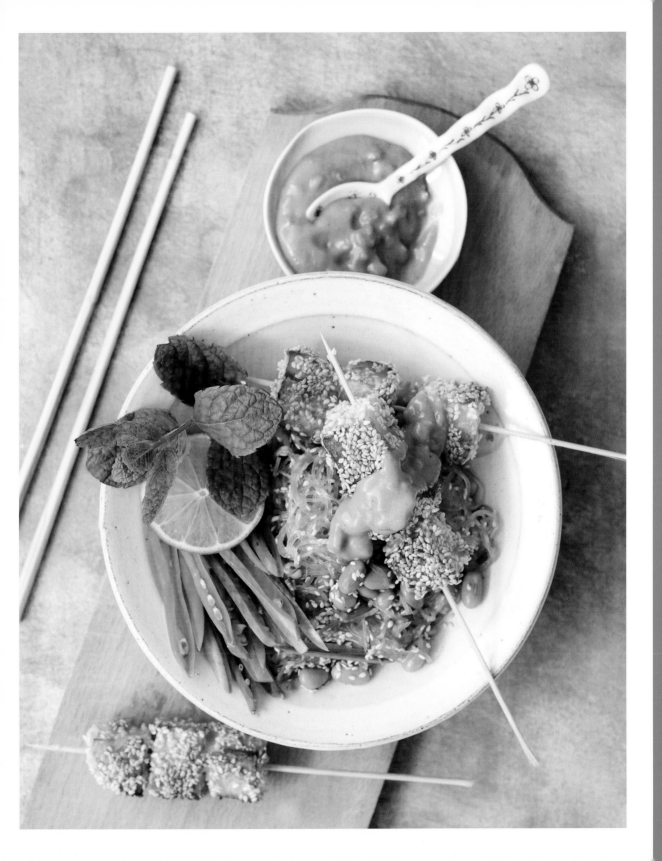

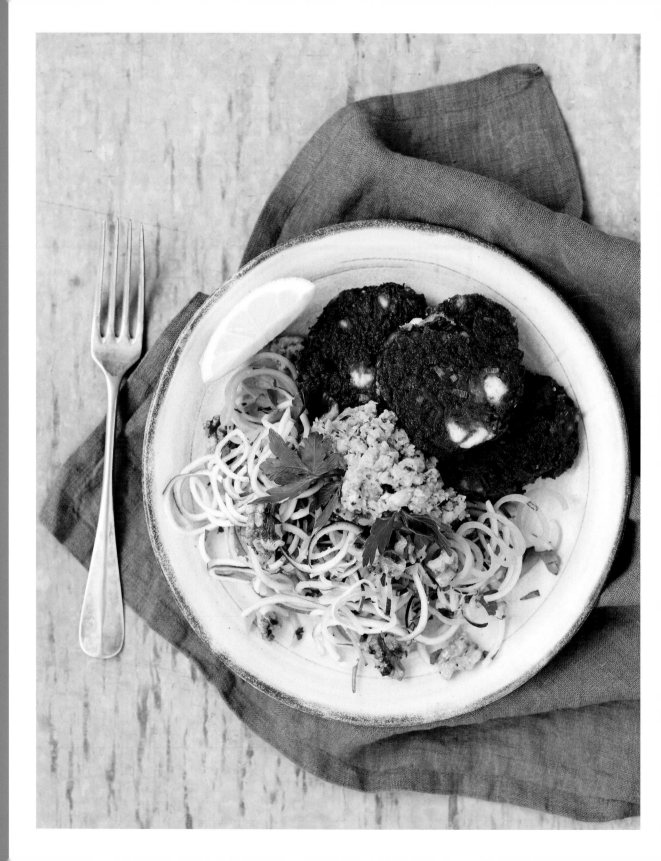

Beet Burgers
WITH FETA CHEESE

*The very best beet burgers! The feta cheese makes them especially tasty,
so my tip to you is to make many of them and freeze them for later.*

475 CALORIES/SERVES 4

1 pound (450 g) peeled and coarsely grated beets

1¾ ounces (½ dl) finely chopped leek—approximately 1¾ inch (5 cm)

5¼ ounces (150 g) crumbled feta cheese

2 eggs

1 cup (2½ dl) oat flour

1 teaspoon salt

½ teaspoon persillade [chopped garlic and parsley]

2 tablespoons olive oil, for frying

Lemon wedges, for garnish

Apple salad

1 apple

1 carrot

½ zucchini

1¾ ounces (½ dl) chopped fresh parsley

Juice from ½ lemon

1¾ ounces (½ dl) chopped, roasted walnuts

1. Preheat the oven to 350°F (175°C). In a bowl, mix all the ingredients for the burgers, except for the olive oil.

2. Heat some olive oil in a skillet. Form the mixture into burgers, and add to the skillet. Brown the burgers until they are nicely browned, about 2 minutes on each side.

3. Place the burgers in an ovenproof dish and leave the burgers in the oven for about 10 minutes.

4. Spiralize or julienne apple, carrot, and zucchini for the apple salad, and place them in a bowl. Mix in parsley, lemon juice, and walnuts.

5. Place the burgers and salad on plates, garnish with lemon wedges, and serve.

Green Quinoa Salad
WITH GOAT CHEESE AND PISTACHIOS

Mixed broccoli turns this salad a lovely shade of green. And mixing it with avocado, apple, and goat cheese makes it even greater, if such a thing were possible!

950 CALORIES/SERVES 2

6 ¾ ounces (2 dl) white quinoa

½ broccoli stem with florets

Juice from ½ lemon

3⅓ ounces (1 dl) frozen soybeans

1 tablespoon olive oil

Salt

Black pepper

2 tablespoons dill, chopped

1 avocado

1 apple

1 stalk celery

1 ounce (30 g) mâche lettuce

7 ounces (200 g) goat cheese

1¾ ounce (½ dl) pistachios, chopped, for garnish

Pea shoots, for garnish

Lemon wedges, for garnish

1. Cook the quinoa following the instructions on the package, about 13 minutes. Drain off the water.
2. Cut the broccoli into florets. Place them in a food processor and mix them fine. Place the broccoli mix in a bowl. Stir in quinoa, lemon juice, soybeans, oil, salt, pepper, and dill.
3. Halve the avocado and the apple. Slice one half of each fruit and save for garnish. Cut the other halves into small chunks. Julienne the celery and then add it to the bowl.
4. Divide the mâche lettuce on the plates and place the quinoa salad on top. Slice the goat cheese and place it on the plates together with the pistachios. Garnish with avocado slices, apple slices, pea shoots, and lemon wedges.

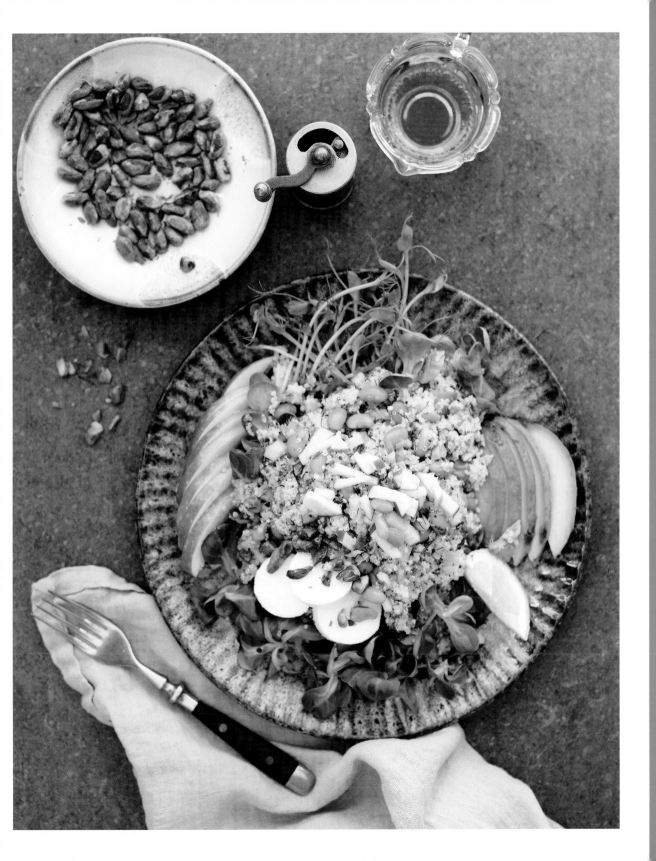

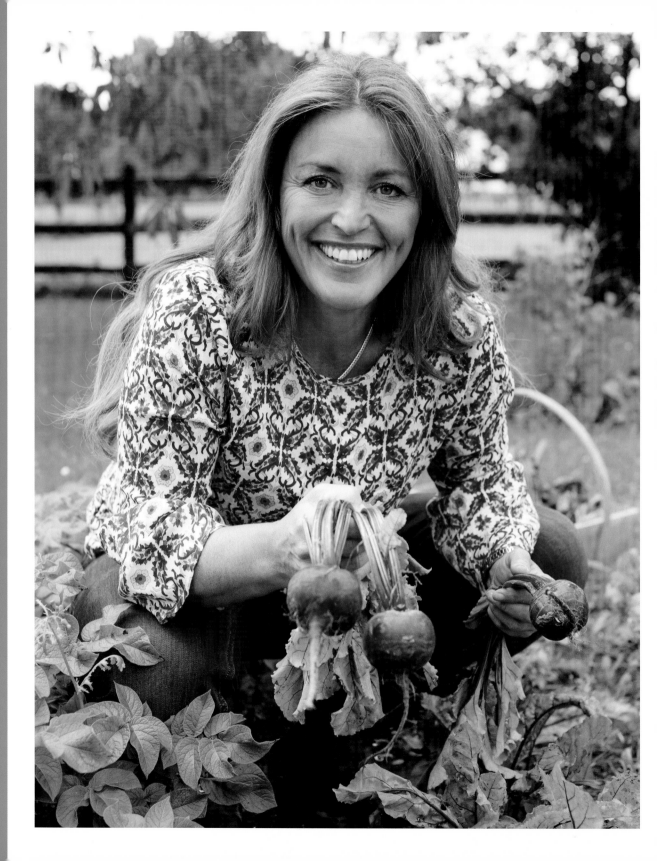

VEGETARIAN
Meal Schedule

DURATION: 2 WEEKS
WEIGHT LOSS: 4½ TO 6½ POUNDS (2–3 KG)

Welcome to my vegetarian kickstart! It's never a bad thing to get some inspiration for recipes whether you have been a vegetarian for many years or if you are simply curious about vegetarian dishes. Here I'll offer you just that—easy, flavorful dishes which are good for your health!

This meal schedule is set up to last two weeks, and is based on a low-carbohydrate diet combined with fast days during which you will eat less than 500 calories. The calorie intake varies a lot from day to day (from about 500 to around 2,000), which gives the metabolism a real push.

You will skip breakfast two days a week and eat your first meal around midday. Those days end with a last meal around 8 p.m. This way of eating is called 16:8 and means that you fast for sixteen hours, followed by an eight-hour eating window. This is another effective weight-loss method and it is very healthy for you.

If you're looking to lose weight, then I suggest that you follow the meal schedule to the letter, and only eat what is included in it. If you don't have any excess weight to lose, you can add on calories by increasing the portion sizes or add in some healthy snacks.

The dishes are simple to prepare, and I have arranged the meal schedule so that on certain days you will eat leftovers and won't have to spend all your time in the kitchen. The dishes keep perfectly in the refrigerator for a few days.

Begin each morning with a big glass of lemon water and ginger: 1¼ cup (3 dl) water, juice of ¼ lemon, and one (1) teaspoon of grated ginger. You can prepare the lemon water in the evening and leave it overnight in the refrigerator.

Drink lots of water during the day—at least 2 quarts (2 liters).

DAY	BREAKFAST	LUNCH	DINNER
Monday **494 calories**	Coffe/tea and lemon water	Carrot Soup with Ginger, p. 82 (150 calories)	Sprouted Buckwheat Salad, Ajvar Pepper Relish, and Feta Cheese, p. 88 (344 calories)
Tuesday **862 calories**	Soy Yogurt with Berries and Mango, p. 74 (174 calories)	Sprouted Buckwheat Salad, Ajvar Pepper Relish, and Feta Cheese (344 calories), *leftovers*	Sliced Vegetable in a Pesto Gratin, p. 91 (370 calories)
Wednesday **470 calories**	Coffee/tea and lemon water	Sliced Vegetable in a Pesto Gratin (370 calories), *leftovers*	Vegetarian Kelp Soup with Tofu, p. 122 (100 calories)
Thursday **1,063 calories**	½ cup (1 dl) soy yogurt (42 calories) with ¼ cup Oat Granola, p. 115 (140 calories)	Carrot Soup with Ginger (150 calories), *leftovers*	Lentil Salad with Halloumi and Carrot Burgers, p. 92 (731 calories)
Friday **1,441 calories**	1 slice Sprouted Bread with Apricots, p. 79 (192 calories) + 1 teaspoon butter, 1 ounce cheese, and bell pepper (129 calories)	Lentil Salad with Halloumi and Carrot Burgers (731 calories), *leftovers*	Italian Cauliflower Pizza, p. 95 (389 calories)
Saturday **1,935 calories**	Pomegranate Beverage with Melon and Almonds, p. 72 (426 calories) (Leftovers must be kept refrigerated!)	Italian Cauliflower Pizza (389 calories), *leftovers*	Spaghetti Pomodoro with Buffalo Mozzarella, p. 97 (850 calories), 1 glass wine (105 calories), Chocolate Crisp with Quinoa, p. 186 (165 calories)
Sunday **1,837 calories**	Pomegranate Beverage with Melon and Almonds (426 calories), *leftovers*	Marinated Chioggia Beets with Feta Cheese, p. 80 (561 calories)	Spaghetti Pomodoro with Buffalo Mozzarella (850 calories), *leftovers*

DAY	BREAKFAST	LUNCH	DINNER
Monday **485 calories**	Coffee/tea and lemon water	Broccoli and Spinach Soup with Halloumi, p. 161 (285 calories)	Rice Wraps with Mango and Curry Sauce, p. 40 (200 calories)
Tuesday **1,563 calories**	½ cup (1 dl) soy yogurt (42 calories) with ¼ cup (½ dl) Oat Granola, p. 115 (140 calories)	Marinated Chioggia Beets with Feta Cheese (561 calories), *leftovers*	Quinoa Salad with Three Cheeses, p. 99 (820 calories)
Wednesday **484 calories**	Coffee/tea and lemon water	Rice Wraps with Mango and Curry Sauce (200 calories), *leftovers*	Broccoli and Spinach Soup with Halloumi (285 calories), *leftovers*
Thursday **2,091 calories**	1 slice Sprouted Bread with Apricots, p. 79 (192 calories) + 1 teaspoon butter, 1 ounce cheese, and bell pepper (129 calories)	Quinoa Salad with Three Cheeses (820 calories), *leftovers*	Sesame Seed–Coated Turnip Skewers with Noodle Salad, p.100 (950 calories)
Friday **1,500 calories**	Chocolate Smoothie Bowl with Chia Seeds, p. 76 (300 calories)	Strawberries with Buffalo Mozzarella and Pistachio Pesto, p. 85 (750 calories)	Halloumi Burgers with Ajvar Pepper Relish, p. 86 (450 calories)
Saturday **1,887 calories**	Red Blueberry Dream Smoothie, p. 148 (322 calories) (Leftovers must be kept refrigerated!)	Halloumi Burgers with Ajvar Pepper Relish (450 calories), *leftovers* Beet Cake with Saffron Crème, p. 189 (535 calories) *or* Roasted Snacks, p. 196 (135 calories + (290 calories)	Beet Burgers with Feta Cheese, p.103 (475 calories) + 1 glass wine (15 cl) (105 calories)
Sunday **1,747 calories**	Red Blueberry Dream Smoothie (322 calories), *leftovers*	Beet Burgers with Feta Cheese (475 calories), *leftovers*	Green Quinoa Salad with Goat Cheese and Pistachios, p. 104 (950 calories)

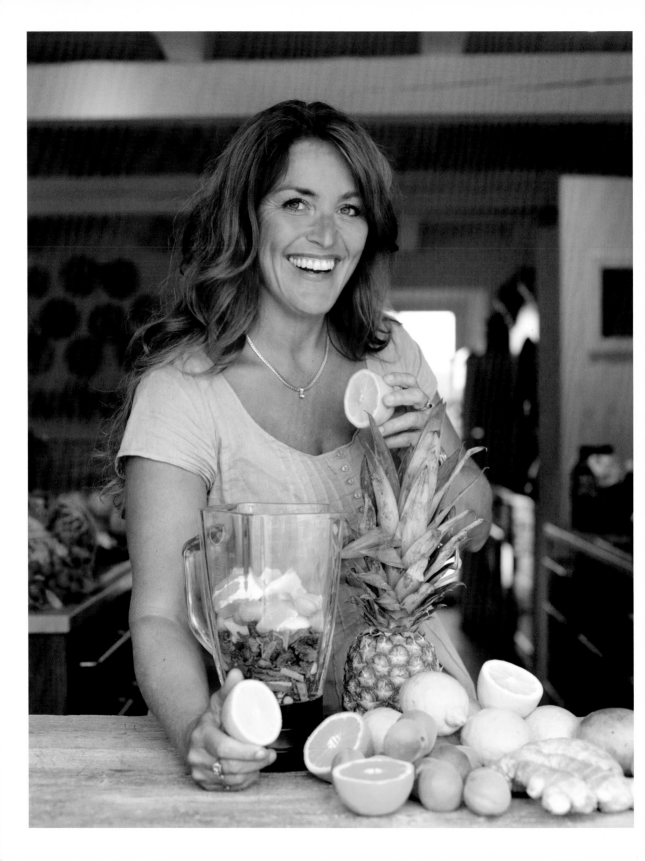

- KICKSTART -
RAW VEGAN
- RECIPES AND MEAL SCHEDULE -

Now we're going to try a week of mixed raw foods and veganism! These dishes are based on a low-carbohydrate diet featuring vegetables and fruits in all the colors of the rainbow. The recipes are free of gluten, refined sugar, cow's milk, and animal protein. You are going to eat a natural and health-giving diet and enjoy many raw food dishes.

Raw foods are raw ingredients that have not been heated much, including raw vegetables of all kinds. Vegetables can be heated to 110°F (42°C) before they begin losing their important digestive enzymes and antioxidants. When you prepare raw foods, the ingredients should be heated as little as possible, or not at all. Stir-fry or steam the vegetables quickly and lightly (but never allow them to go over 110°F [42°C]). Do not allow the food's temperature to rise above 120°F (70°C) to ensure that you'll be able to reap maximum benefit from the minerals and vitamins.

Raw foods provide many other health benefits, such as high fiber content that makes you feel full (which exercises the intestines); a great intake of enzymes that aid digestion; and chewing satisfaction that ensures that you masticate your food longer, which also helps to promote good digestive health.

In this kickstart, I also want to inspire you to try out vegan dishes—vegetarian meals free of all animal foods, like eggs, cheese, and milk.

I have witnessed many who claim that they feel a sense of lightness after one week of this nutrition. Not just the actual lightness due to weight loss, but maybe an all-over feeling of lightness in both body and mind. So this might be just the thing in your future for improving your health!

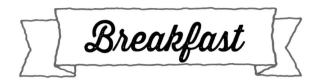

SLIM-DOWN
Raspberry Drink

Cranberry powder is tart and tasty, and can be used in smoothies or mixed directly into water. Cranberries contain lots of antioxidants, primarily flavonoids.

51 CALORIES/MAKES 6 SMALL SERVINGS

Juice from 3 oranges
Juice from 1 lime
2 tablespoons fresh grated ginger
2 tablespoons cranberry powder
7 ounces (200 g) raspberries, frozen
Sprigs of mint
Approximately 1¼ cups (3 dl) cold water

1. Mix all the ingredients in a blender to a smooth mixture. Add more water if necessary.
2. Serve in shot glasses to start the day with an antioxidant boost. Store the drink in the refrigerator in a closed bottle. Keeps for about 3 to 4 days.

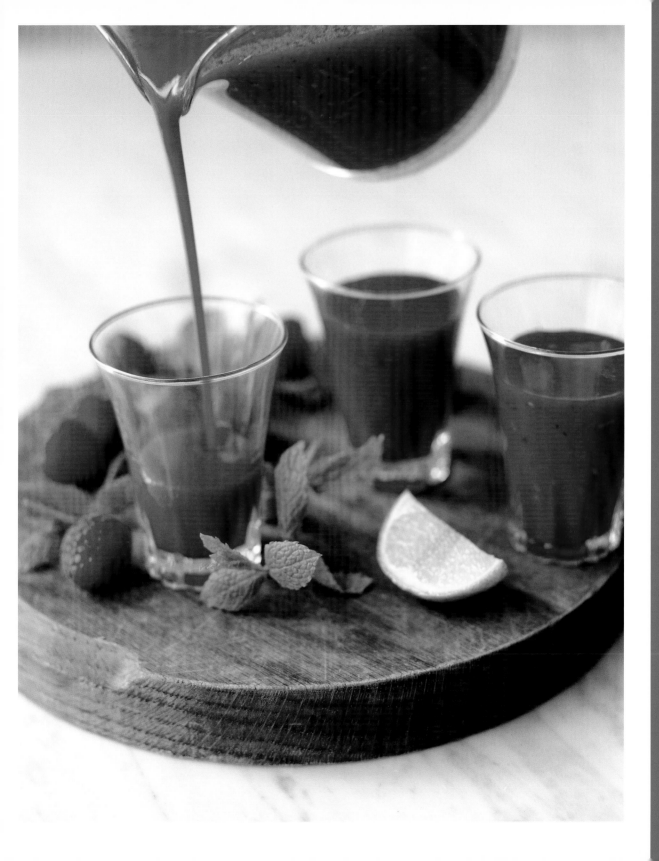

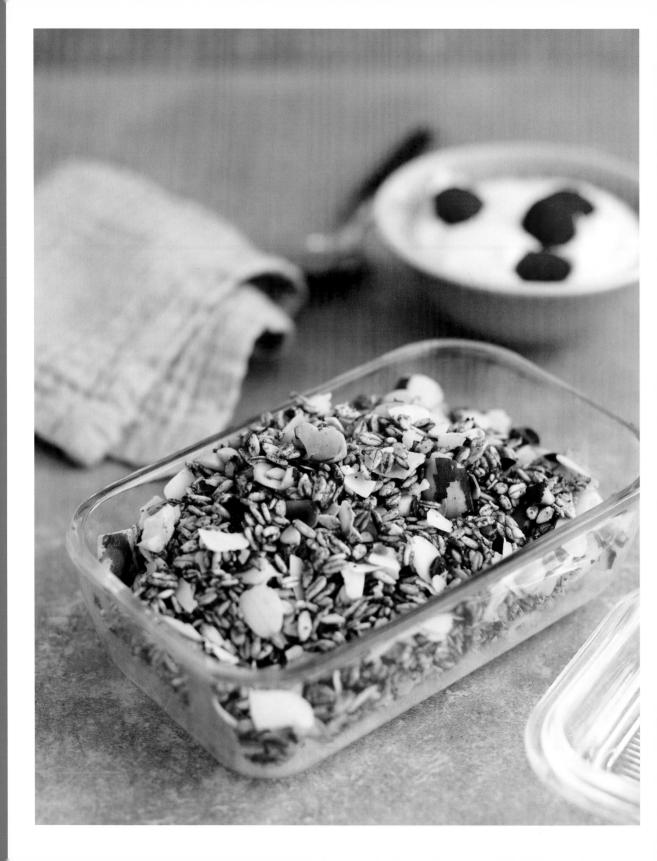

Oat Granola

Roasted oat groats and nuts infuse a delicious and filling flavor to this crunchy granola along with lots of chewing satisfaction. And why not try it heated up a little? Sooo good!

140 CALORIES/(1 SERVING = 4 TABLESPOONS/1/4 DL) **– MAKES APPROXIMATELY 15 SERVINGS**

6¾ ounces (2 dl) Brazil nuts

3⅓ ounces (1 dl) slivered almonds

1¼ cups (3 dl) oat groats

1 teaspoon cinnamon, ground

½ teaspoon cardamom, ground

2 tablespoons honey

3⅓ ounces (1 dl) coconut, grated

1. Chop the Brazil nuts coarsely and roast them along with the slivered almonds and oat groats for a few minutes in a dry skillet, stirring frequently.
2. Sprinkle with cinnamon and cardamom and drizzle with the honey. Stir for about a minute and then remove from the heat when the granola has taken on a bit of color.
3. Pour the granola into a bowl or jar with a lid and add the coconut flakes. Let cool completely and put on the lid.

Buckwheat Porridge

WITH DRIED FRUIT AND SEEDS

When I'm craving porridge (which happens quite often), I happily turn to this recipe. This porridge isn't just very tasty—it also keeps me satiated for a long time.

533 CALORIES/SERVES 2

3⅓ ounces (1 dl) buckwheat

1 cup (2½ dl) water

1 pinch salt

1 teaspoon honey

1 teaspoon cinnamon, ground

1¾ ounces (½ dl) sunflower seeds

1¾ ounces (½ dl) pumpkin seeds

2 tablespoons flaxseed

3½ ounces (100 g) mixed dried fruit, chopped

Almond milk, for serving

Topping

Slivered almonds
Pumpkin seeds
Ground cinnamon

1. Rinse the crushed buckwheat in boiling water (see information about rinsing on p. 88) and let it drain.
2. Place all porridge ingredients except almond milk in a saucepan. Bring to a boil and then let it simmer on low heat for about 7 minutes. Dilute with more water if necessary.
3. Pour the porridge into a bowl and top it with slivered almonds, pumpkin seeds, and ground cinnamon. Serve with almond milk.

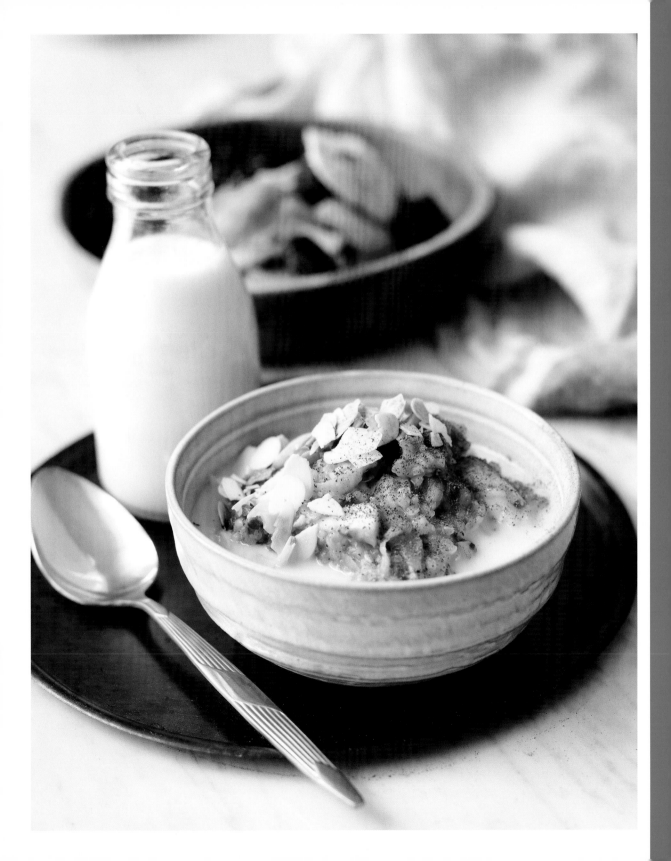

Smoothie Bowl with Mango

Equally good as breakfast or a dessert. Or at any time of the day, for that matter.

293 CALORIES/SERVES 1

6¾ ounces (2 dl) diced
  frozen mango
6¾ fluid ounces (2 dl)
  coconut milk
Grated peel from ½
  lemon + extra for
  sprinkling
⅕ teaspoon (1 krm)
  vanilla powder

Topping

½ fresh mango, sliced
2 tablespoons chopped
  pistachios
2 tablespoons coconut
  flakes

1. Place frozen mango, coconut milk, lemon peel,
   and vanilla powder in a food processor and mix
   to a smooth texture.
2. Pour the mixture into a bowl and top it with
   fresh mango, pistachios, coconut flakes, and
   some grated lemon peel.

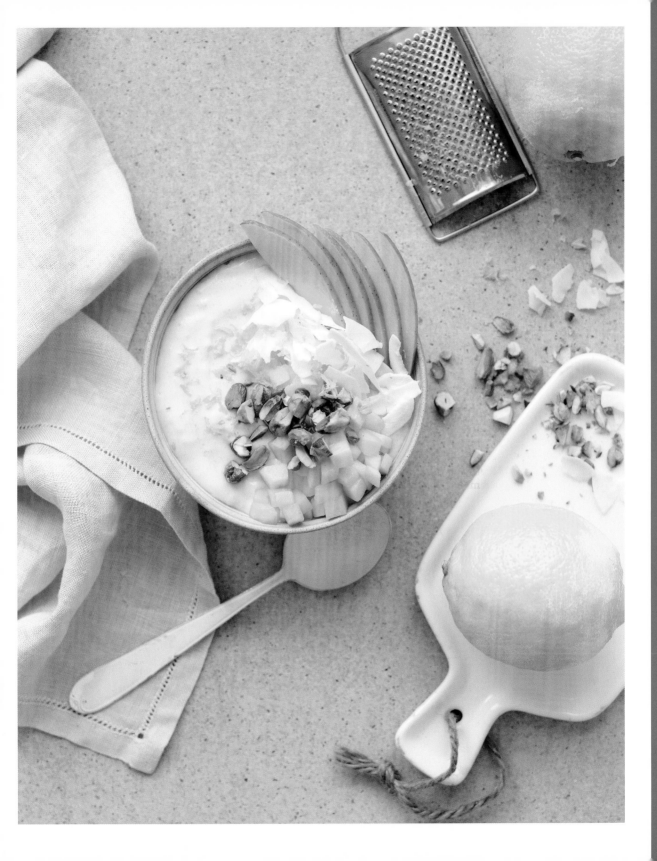

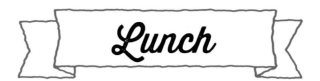

Cauliflower Soup
WITH ROASTED CHICKPEAS

A silky smooth soup with an exciting topping.

232 CALORIES/SERVES 4

1 yellow onion
1 clove garlic
1 tablespoon olive oil
1 medium cauliflower
3¼ cups (8 dl) water
1½ teaspoons organic,
   gluten-free stock
   powder
3⅓ ounces (1 dl)
   pecorino cheese,
   grated
Salt
Black pepper

Topping

1 can (14 ounces or
   400 g) chickpeas
1 teaspoon honey
Salt
Mediterranean herbs
1 stalk celery
Fresh chervil leaves

1. Chop the onion and garlic. Heat the olive oil in a large saucepan and fry the onion and garlic for a few minutes. Separate the cauliflower into smaller florets and place them in the saucepan—save a few florets for frying and use as topping. Add water and stock powder and bring to a boil. Let simmer until the cauliflower is soft, about 10 minutes.

2. In a blender, mix the soup until smooth and pour it back into the saucepan. Add the cheese and let it melt. Stir occasionally and season with salt and black pepper. Keep the soup warm.

3. Rinse the chickpeas with cold water. Let them drain thoroughly and then roast them, while stirring, in a dry skillet for a few minutes together with honey, salt, and herbs. Finely julienne the celery. Thinly slice the saved cauliflower florets. Fry them in a teaspoon of oil until they are nicely colored.

4. Divide the soup between bowls and top with chickpeas, celery, fried cauliflower, and chervil.

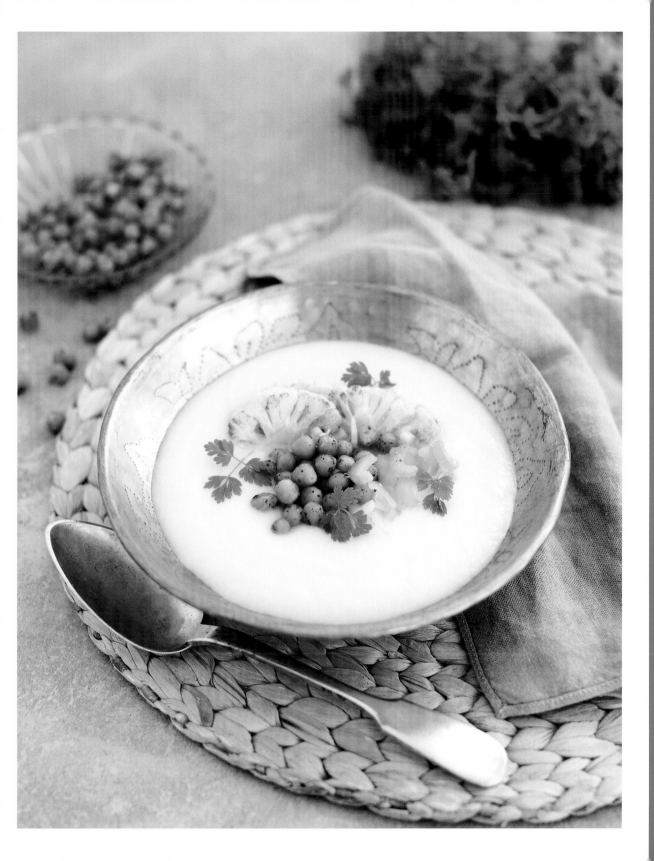

Vegan Kelp Soup
WITH TOFU

A flavorful soup that provides energy and nutrition. Vary it by using your favorite vegetables and what you already have at home.

100 CALORIES/SERVES 4

2 cups (5 dl) water
1 tablespoon stock powder
1 tablespoon kecap manis sweet soy sauce
½ red chili, finely chopped
1 tablespoon fresh grated ginger
1 small clove garlic, finely chopped
Juice from ½ lemon
2 teaspoons sesame oil
10 mushrooms
1¾-inch (5 cm) leek
2 stalks of celery
1 carrot
⅔ ounce (20 g) dried kelp
Salt
Black pepper
3½ ounces (100 g) marinated tofu
1 bunch fresh cilantro, for garnish
2 tablespoons chopped chives, for garnish

1. In a large saucepan, bring the water, stock powder, and soy sauce to a boil. Add the chili, ginger, garlic, lemon juice, and sesame oil. Let simmer for a few minutes.
2. Slice the mushrooms. Julienne the leek and celery. Peel and slice the carrot fine. Place everything in the saucepan along with the kelp. Season with salt and pepper. Let simmer for 2 minutes.
3. Dice the tofu and coarsely chop the cilantro leaves—leave a few for garnish. Stir it all into the soup before serving. Serve the soup in deep bowls and top with chopped chives and cilantro.

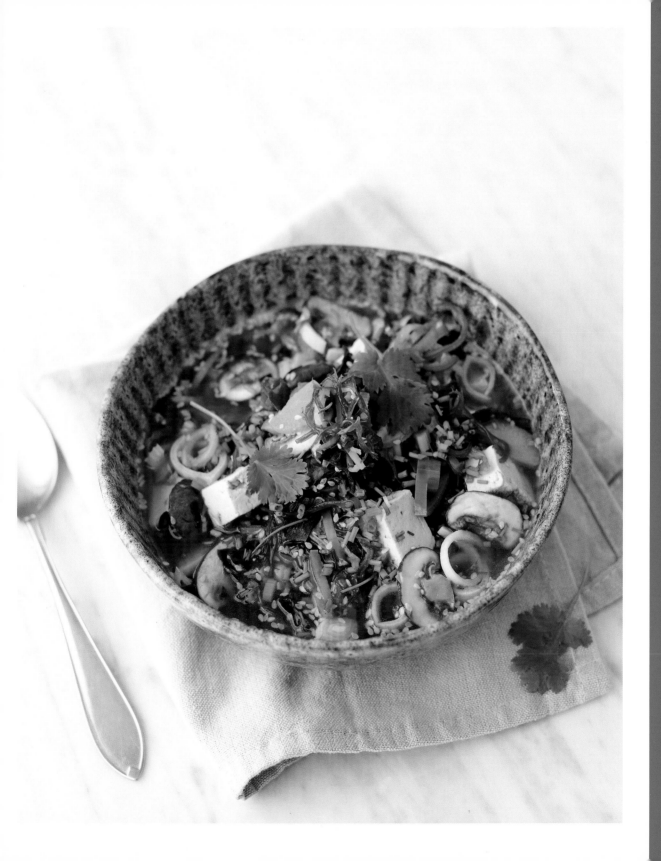

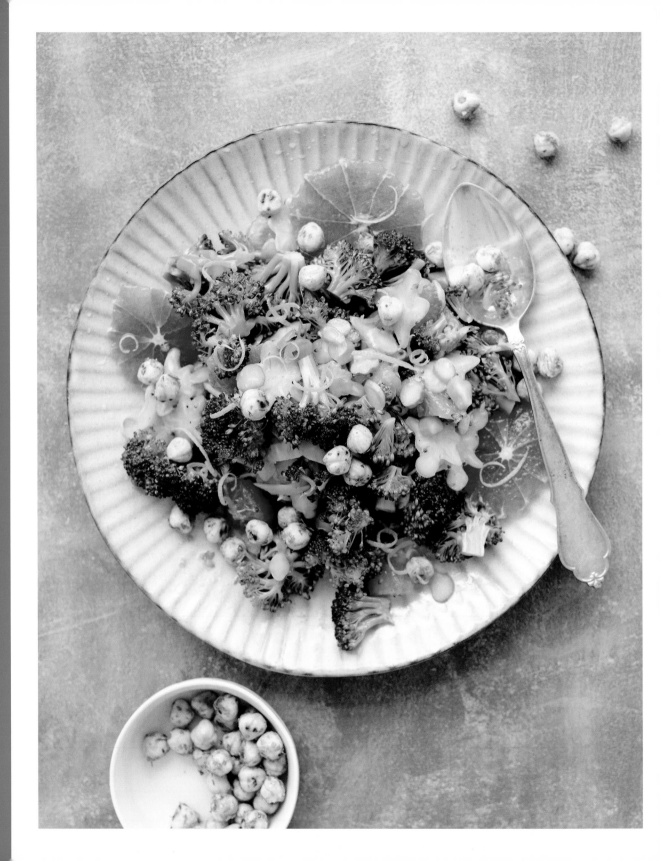

Lemon-Marinated Broccoli
WITH GRAPEFRUIT

Crunchy and good-for-you broccoli with a crisp lemon flavor.
A true taste sensation with the tarragon-roasted hazelnuts!

407 CALORIES/SERVES 2

1 head broccoli
½ lemon
1 tablespoon olive oil
Salt
Black pepper
1 grapefruit

Tarragon-roasted
hazelnuts (filberts)

3⅓ ounces (1 dl)
  hazelnuts/filberts,
  without skins
1 teaspoon honey
⅕ teaspoon (1 krm)
  dried French tarragon
Salt flakes

1. Separate the broccoli into florets and finely slice the stem. Put it all in a bowl.
2. Cut off the yellow outer layer on the lemon and grate it fine, or use a zester. Put the zest aside for the moment. Press the lemon juice over the broccoli and drizzle with olive oil. Season with salt and black pepper and stir thoroughly.
3. Cut off the grapefruit peel with a sharp knife. Cut a few thin slices from the grapefruit and cut fine segments from the rest. Add the segments to the bowl and divide the broccoli salad between the plates.
4. Place the hazelnuts in a dry skillet over high heat. Roast while stirring for a few minutes and then stir in honey, tarragon, and salt.
5. Sprinkle the freshly roasted hazelnuts over the broccoli and garnish with lemon strips and grapefruit slices.

Tuscan Black Cabbage Salad
WITH DILL, HALLOUMI, AND POMEGRANATE

Black and green kales are hearty cabbage varieties that offer a lot of chewing satisfaction and wonderful flavors. Plus you'll get loads of nutrients!

350 CALORIES/SERVES 2

Dressing

1 teaspoon honey
1 tablespoon apple cider vinegar
1 tablespoon olive oil
1 tablespoon strong, sweet mustard
1¾ ounce (½ dl) fresh dill, chopped + extra for garnish
Salt
Black pepper

Salad

7 ounces (200 g) black cabbage or kale
½ red onion
Pomegranate seeds from ½ a fruit
1 tablespoon sunflower seed
1 teaspoon olive oil
2⅔ ounces (75 gr) halloumi, sliced

1. Start by stirring together all the dressing ingredients in a bowl.
2. Julienne the cabbage and the red onion. Add it all to the bowl and massage the cabbage for a few minutes. Place the mixture on plates and sprinkle with pomegranate seeds.
3. Heat a dry skillet and roast the sunflower seeds for a minute or two while stirring. Sprinkle the seeds over the salad.
4. Add oil to the skillet and fry the halloumi slices on both sides. Top the salad with the cheese and some chopped dill and serve immediately.

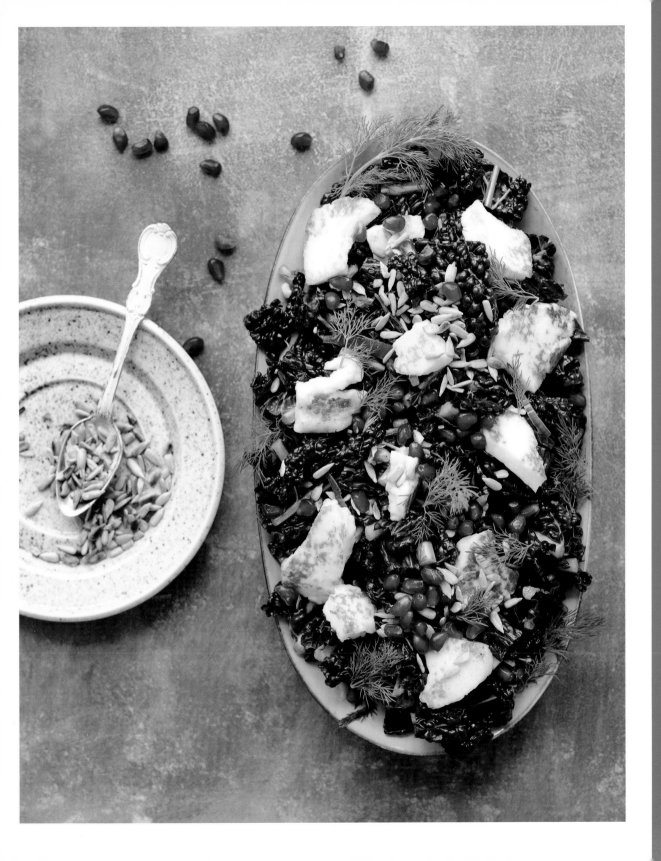

Stir-fried Vegetables
WITH KELP NOODLES

Kelp noodles are low in calories and have hardly any carbohydrates. They're also quickly prepared with a wonderful consistency. Here we've seasoned them with an Asian marinade.

350 CALORIES/SERVES 2

Topping

2 tablespoons cashews
Salt
1 teaspoon honey

5¼ ounces (150 g) kelp noodles
Approximately 3½ ounces (100 g) fresh mini corn cobs
1¾ ounces (50 g) fresh sugar snap peas
1 carrot
1 salad onion
1 red bell pepper
½ mango
1 teaspoon canola oil
1 teaspoon fresh grated ginger
1 small clove garlic, grated
½ red chili, finely chopped

1 teaspoon sesame oil
1 tablespoon kecap manis sweet soy sauce
4 tablespoons teriyaki sauce
Juice from ½ lime
Salt
White pepper
3 tablespoons fresh cilantro, chopped

1. Start with the topping. Heat a dry skillet and roast the cashews for a few minutes. Sprinkle with some salt and drizzle with the honey.
2. Rinse the noodles in cold water. Slice the mini corn cobs and the sugar snap peas lengthwise. Peel and thinly slice the carrot lengthwise. Julienne the salad onion and bell pepper. Cut the mango into smaller pieces.
3. Heat the canola oil in a wok or skillet and fry the ginger, garlic, chili, sesame oil, mini corn cobs, carrot, bell pepper, and mango for a few minutes while stirring.
4. Stir in the kecap manis , teriyaki sauce, lime juice, seaweed noodles, and sugar snap peas, and let it warm up. Season with salt and pepper. Sprinkle with salad onion, cilantro, and roasted nuts.

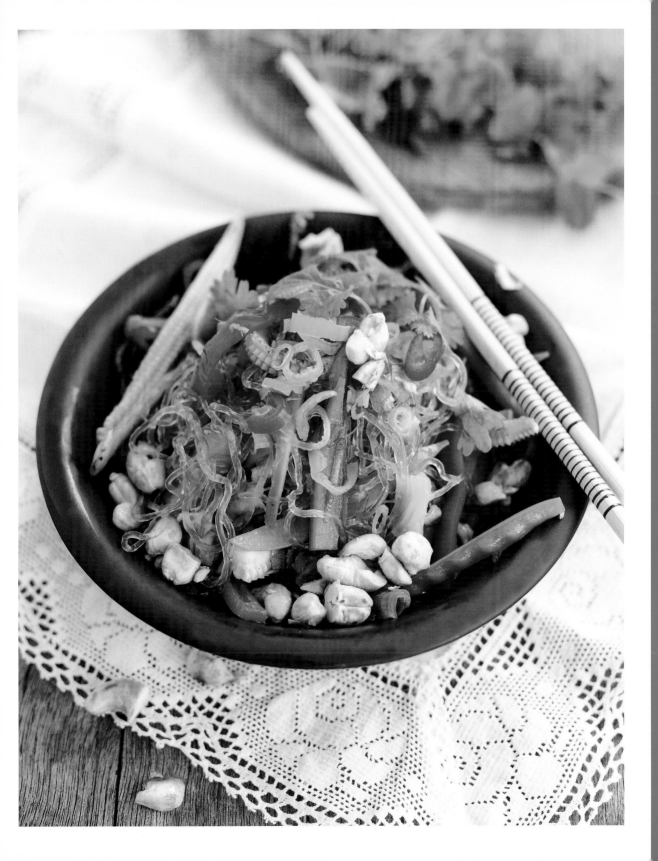

Rice Wraps
WITH PEANUT SAUCE

Fresh Asian-inspired wraps with vegetables and peanuts—perfect for brown bagging or to serve guests!

425 CALORIES/SERVES 4

Peanut sauce

3⅓ ounces (100 g) unsweetened peanut butter

2 tablespoons soy sauce

1¾ fluid ounces (½ dl) water

3⅓ fluid ounces (1 dl) coconut cream

Salt

Black pepper

Wraps

1 carrot

1 avocado

1 mango

3½ ounces (100 g) sugar snap peas

1 salad onion

12 rice papers

3⅓ ounces (1 dl) red cabbage, julienned

½ bunch fresh cilantro

Garnish

3⅓ ounces (1 dl) salt peanuts

2 limes cut into wedges

1. Make the peanut sauce first. Mix all the ingredients in a saucepan and heat while stirring until the sauce is smooth. Put aside.
2. Cut the carrot into thin slices. Peel the avocado and mango and remove the pits. Cut the fruits into thin sticks. Finely julienne the sugar snap peas and salad onion.
3. Soak a rice paper in a plate with cold water. Remove the paper when it feels soft—about 20 seconds—and place it on a cutting board. Place a little bit of all the vegetables in the center of the rice paper, top with cilantro, and roll it into a wrap. Repeat the procedure with the remaining papers.
4. Place the wraps on plates, drizzle with peanut sauce, and sprinkle with chopped peanuts. Garnish with lime wedges.

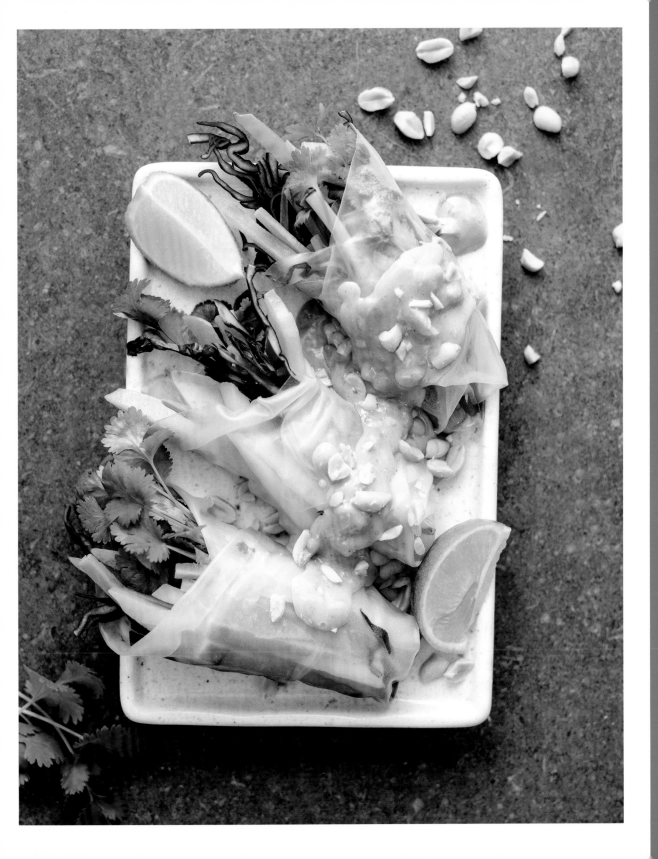

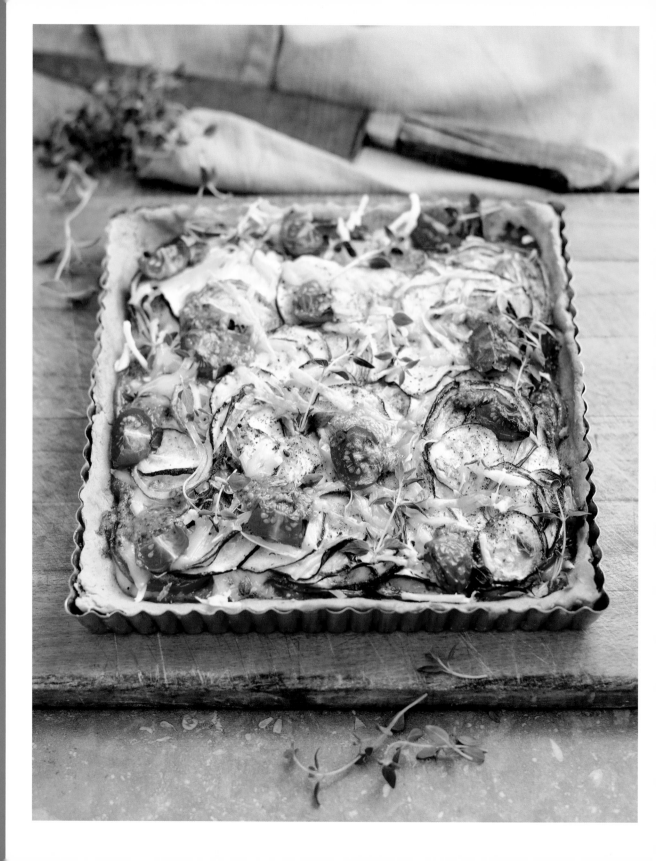

VEGAN
Chickpea Pie

The perfect pie to bring to the table or to cut into portions and freeze for future brown bag lunches. A green salad makes a nice side.

400 CALORIES/SERVES 4

Pastry

2 cans chickpeas, each 14 ounces (400 g)
½ teaspoon salt
2 tablespoons unsweetened peanut butter
1 tablespoon oat flour
1 tablespoon buckwheat flour
1 tablespoon coconut oil

Filling

3⅓ fluid ounces (1 dl) ajvar relish
2 tomatoes
½ zucchini
½ red onion
7 ounces (200 g) vegan cheese, grated
1¾ fluid ounces (½ dl) green pesto (see p. 58 or use store bought) + some extra for garnish
Salt
Black pepper
Mediterranean herbs
1 tablespoon olive oil
6 cherry tomatoes
Fresh thyme, for garnish

1. Preheat the oven to 300°F (150°C). Rinse the chickpeas for the pastry in water, let them drain, and place them in a food processor. Add the rest of the pastry ingredients and mix to make smooth dough.

2. Flatten the dough into a springform pan, about 9¾ x 9¾ inches (25 cm x 25 cm). Prick the bottom with a fork and prebake the pastry for about 25 minutes. Increase the heat to 400°F (200°C).

3. Spread ajvar relish over the bottom of the pie. Slice tomatoes, zucchini, and onion and layer them together with cheese and pesto. Season with salt, pepper, and herbs and drizzle with olive oil. Cut the tomatoes into wedges and scatter them over the pie.

4. Bake in the middle of the oven for about 20 minutes. Garnish with thyme and dot on the pesto.

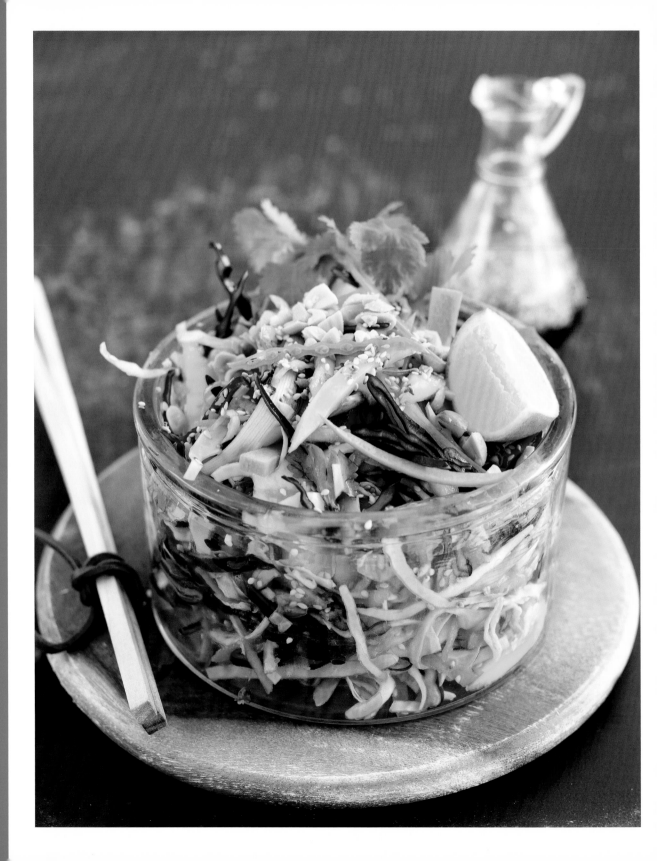

ASIAN RAW
Food Salad

Lots of chewing satisfaction and exciting flavors.
A salad that fills you up for a long time.

525 CALORIES/SERVES 2

Dressing

1¾ ounces (½ dl) white
  sesame seeds
½ tablespoon fresh
  ginger, grated
1 tablespoon sesame oil
2 tablespoons soy sauce
1 teaspoon honey
1 tablespoon sweet
  chili sauce
Juice from ½ lime

Salad

2 cups (5 dl) mixed red
  and white cabbage,
  julienned
1 carrot
1 avocado
1 mango
3⅓ ounces (100 g)
  sugar snap peas
½ bunch fresh cilantro

Garnish

Wedges of ½ lime
Fresh cilantro leaves
1 tablespoon salted
  peanuts

1. Start by making the dressing. Roast the sesame seeds in a dry, hot skillet. In a bowl, mix the rest of the dressing ingredients and set aside.

2. Place the cabbage in a bowl. Cut the carrot into thin strips and add to the bowl with the cabbage. Peel the avocado and mango and remove the pits. Cut the fruits in thin strips. Julienne the sugar snap peas lengthwise. Chop the cilantro leaves. Mix everything together in the bowl.

3. Drizzle dressing over the salad and garnish with lime wedges, cilantro, and peanuts.

Asian Cauliflower Rice
WITH WASABI NUTS

Grated raw cauliflower with a touch of Asian flavor.
The chopped wasabi nuts provide that little bit of extra punch!

425 CALORIES/SERVES 2

1 small cauliflower
Juice from 1 lime
1 teaspoon canola oil
1 tablespoon sweet
 chili sauce
1 teaspoon fresh grated
 ginger
3⅓ ounces (1 dl)
 soybeans
Salt
Black pepper
1 salad onion
1 red chili
1 mango
Leaves from ½ bunch of
 cilantro
3½ ounces (100 g)
 sugar snap peas
2 large cabbage or
 lettuce leaves
1¾ ounces (½ dl)
 wasabi nuts
Pea shoots, for garnish
Lime wedges, optional

1. Coarsely grate the cauliflower and place it in a bowl. Add the lime juice, oil, and sweet chili sauce and mix thoroughly. Add the ginger, soybeans, salt, and black pepper.

2. Julienne the salad onion and chili. Remove the pit and peel the mango. Set aside a few thin slices of mango and dice the rest of the mango. Chop the cilantro—save a few leaves for the garnish—and julienne the sugar snap peas lengthwise. Mix all of this into the cauliflower rice, but save a few sugar snap peas for garnish.

3. Line two deep bowls with one cabbage leaf each. Place cauliflower rice on top. Coarsely chop the wasabi nuts and sprinkle over the cauliflower rice. Garnish with mango slices, cilantro, sugar snap peas, pea shoots, and maybe a few lime wedges.

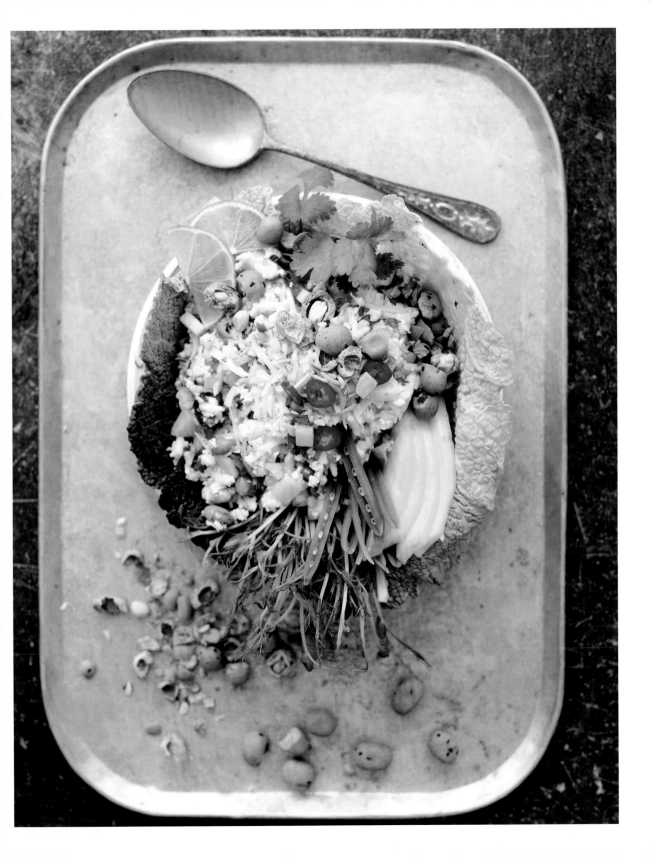

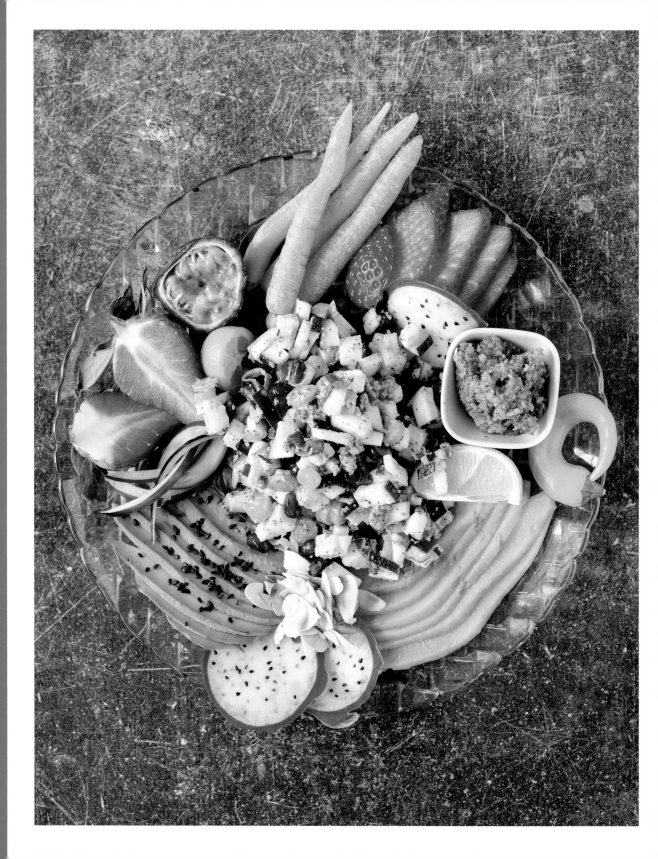

Raw Food Plate
WITH CILANTRO PESTO

Very fresh and delicious, and extra thrilling with the cilantro pesto!
Leftovers can be used with some of the Asian dishes,
like the cauliflower rice on page 136.

630 CALORIES/SERVES 2

Cilantro pesto

Leaves from ½ bunch of cilantro
2½ ounces (¾ dl) almonds
½ clove garlic
3 tablespoons olive oil
Lime or lemon juice, as desired

Pineapple salsa

1 salad onion
1 avocado
¼ fresh pineapple
4-inch (10 cm) hothouse cucumber
1 baby carrot

Raw Food Plate

1 avocado
½ small papaya
4 strawberries
1 dragon fruit
¼ red onion
8 baby carrots
1 passion fruit
2 tablespoons roasted almond slivers
2 tablespoons dried cranberries
½ lime in wedges, for garnish

1. Start by making the cilantro pesto. Place all the pesto ingredients in a food processor and process to make a pesto consistency. Season with citrus juice.

2. Julienne the salad onion for the pineapple salsa and place it in a bowl. Halve and peel the avocado and remove the pit. Peel the pineapple and remove the hard core in the middle. Finely dice avocado, pineapple, cucumber, and carrot and add to the bowl together with half of the pesto. Divide the salsa between 2 plates.

3. Slice the avocado, papaya, strawberries, dragon fruit, and red onion and scatter all around the salsa. Halve the passion fruit and place it on the plates and top with roasted almond slivers and cranberries. Garnish with lime wedges. Serve with the remaining pesto.

Roasted Root Vegetables
WITH BRUSSELS SPROUTS AND POMEGRANATE

A warm salad topped with roasted walnuts and apple. Colorful and exciting!

426 CALORIES/SERVES 2

1 carrot
1 parsnip
½ sweet potato
5¼ ounces (150 g) fresh Brussels sprouts
1 small red onion
1 small clove garlic
1 tablespoon olive oil
Salt
Black pepper
⅕ teaspoon (1 krm) Mediterranean herbs

Topping

3⅓ ounces (1 dl) walnuts, chopped
1 teaspoon honey
Salt
½ red apple
Seeds from ½ pomegranate
2¼ ounces (60 g) fresh spinach leaves

1. Preheat the oven to 450°F (225°C). Dice the root vegetables and place them in a small baking pan.
2. Halve the Brussels sprouts, chop the red onion, and finely chop the garlic clove. Spread it over the baking pan. Drizzle with olive oil and season with salt, pepper, and Mediterranean herbs. Stir the contents. Roast the mixture in the oven for about 20 minutes. Stir the vegetables occasionally.
3. Meanwhile, heat a dry skillet and roast the walnuts for a minute while stirring. Drizzle with honey and season with some salt. Set aside.
4. Slice the apple. Sprinkle the slices and pomegranate seeds over the warm root vegetables and arrange the spinach leaves all around. Sprinkle with nuts and serve.

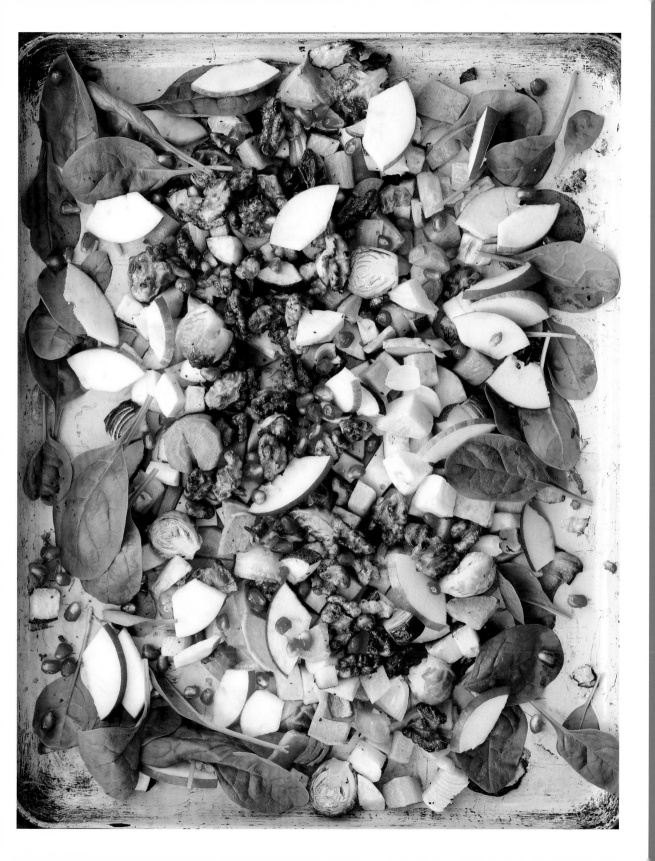

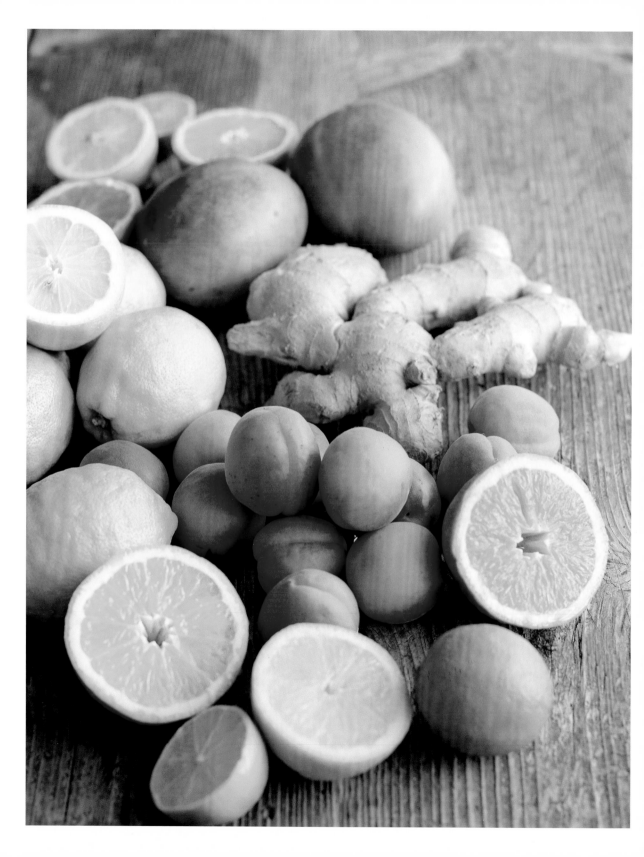

KICKSTART

RAW VEGAN
Meal Schedule

DURATION: 1 WEEK
WEIGHT LOSS: APPROXIMATELY 1¼ POUNDS (2 KG)

Welcome to a week full of raw foods and vegan nutrition! This meal schedule lasts one week and gives you a good look at this way of eating. You can continue to eat like this for another week if you like the dishes, or you can introduce the dishes into your future daily meal routine.

The schedule is based on low-carbohydrate nutrition combined with intermittent fasting when you consume less than 500 calories per day. The calorie intake varies quite a lot from day to day (from about 500 to around 2,000) which gives the metabolism a real jolt.

You'll skip breakfast two days out of the week and instead eat your first meal at around noon. Those days will have their last meals around 8 p.m. This is called 16:8, and means that you fast for sixteen hours and have an eight-hour eating window. This is another very effective weight-loss method that is also very beneficial for your health.

If your goal is weight loss, you will follow the schedule to the letter and only eat what is included in the schedule. If you don't need to lose any weight, go ahead and add more calories by making larger portions or add healthy snacks, like the Sesame Seed Crackers on p. 38 with some of the delicious and flavorful dips on p. 197. Or maybe enjoy some Cashew Balls from p. 194?

The dishes are easy to prepare, and I have arranged the schedule so that on some days you eat leftovers, which ensures that you don't spend all your day in the kitchen. The leftovers keep well in the refrigerator for a few days.

Preferably start each morning with a big glass of lemon water with some added ginger: pour 1 ¼ cup (3 dl) water into a glass and add the juice of ¼ lemon, and add 1 teaspoon of grated ginger. Stir and enjoy!

Continue to drink water throughout the day—around 2 quarts (2 liters) is good.

DAY	BREAKFAST	LUNCH	DINNER
Monday **582 calories**	Coffee/tea and lemon water	Cauliflower Soup with Roasted Chickpeas, p. 120 (232 calories)	Stir-fried Vegetables with Kelp Noodles, p. 128 (350 calories)
Tuesday **928 calories**	3 servings Slim-Down Raspberry Drink, p. 112 (153 calories)	Stir-fried Vegetables with Kelp Noodles, (350 calories) *leftovers*	Rice Wraps with Peanut Sauce, p. 130 (425 calories)
Wednesday **500 calories**	Coffee/tea and lemon water	Vegan Kelp Soup with Tofu, p. 122 (100 calories)	Vegan Chickpea Pie, p. 133 (400 calories)
Thursday **1,114 calories**	½ cup (1 dl) soy yogurt (42 calories) with ¼ cup (½ dl) Oat Granola, p. 115 (140 calories)	Lemon-Marinated Broccoli with Grapefruit, p. 125 (407 calories)	Asian Raw Food Salad with Wasabi Nuts, p. 136 (425 calories)
Friday **1,308 calories**	Buckwheat Porridge with Dried Fruit and Seeds, p. 116 (533 calories)	Tuscan Black Cabbage Salad with Dill, Halloumi, and Pomegranate, p. 126 (350 calories)	Asian Cauliflower Rice with Wasabi Nuts, p. 136 (425 calories)
Saturday **1,894 calories**	Smoothie Bowl with Mango, p. 118 (293 calories)	Asian Cauliflower Rice with Wasabi Nuts (425 calories), *leftovers*	Raw Food Plate with Cilantro Pesto, p. 139 (630 calories), 1 glass of wine (105 calories), Raw mango cake, p. 190 (441 calories) *or* Raw Raspberry and Chocolate Cake, p. 193 (303 calories)
Sunday **1,238 calories**	½ cup (1 dl) soy yogurt (42 calories) with ¼ cup (½ dl) Oat Granola (140 calories)	Raw Food Plate with Cilantro Pesto (630 calories), *leftovers*	Roasted Root Vegetables with Brussels Sprouts and Pomegranate, p. 140 (426 calories)

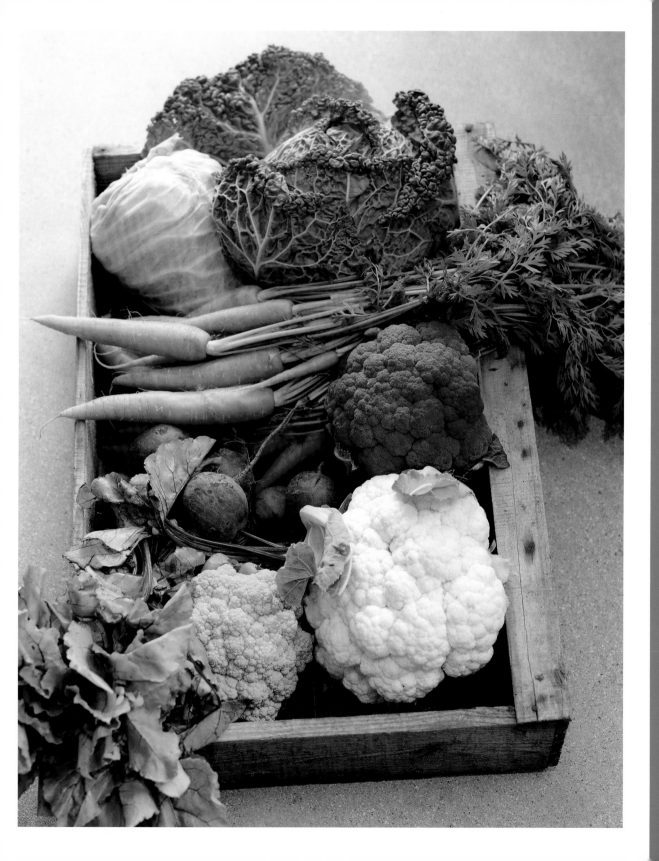

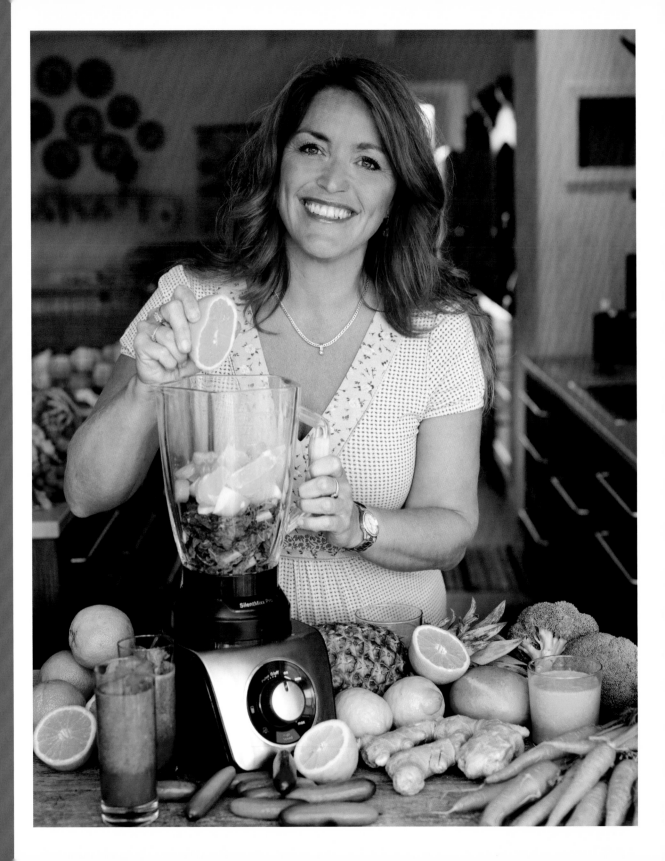

JUICING

Welcome to a world full of healthy and fresh juices that will effectively cleanse your body and give you an amazing energy kick!

By doing a four-day juice fast, you'll cleanse your body of toxins, and you'll oxygenate your cells. Clean out all the free radicals, toxins, and waste products, and boost your body with more vitamins, minerals, and antioxidants than usual. You will feel and see the difference—in body, skin, hair, gut, intestines . . . and your temper.

I recommend that during this kickstart you give yourself a lot of "me" time. Try to go to bed early, sleep extra late, breathe, take a warm bath or a plea-sant sauna. Preferably scrub your skin during these days so it, too, will be cleansed of toxins. Quiet yoga moments or nice nature walks fit in very well during this week—it helps you dust off your brain and ener-gize your blood circulation.

This juice fast will be a new experience, and once finished, you drink the juices for breakfast or as a snack in your new healthy life.

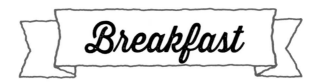

RED BLUEBERRY DREAM
Smoothie

*There are loads of antioxidants in beets and blueberries,
and so there are lots in this smoothie!*

322 CALORIES/SERVES 2

1 fresh beet
1 orange
**8 ounces (225 g)
blueberries, frozen**
**Seeds from 1
pomegranate**
2 cups (5 dl) water

1. Peel the beet and the orange. Cut them into pieces and place in a blender together with the rest of the ingredients (preferably save a few pomegranate seeds for garnish).
2. Blend to make a smoothie and pour into a glass or a bottle. Garnish with pomegranate seeds when serving.

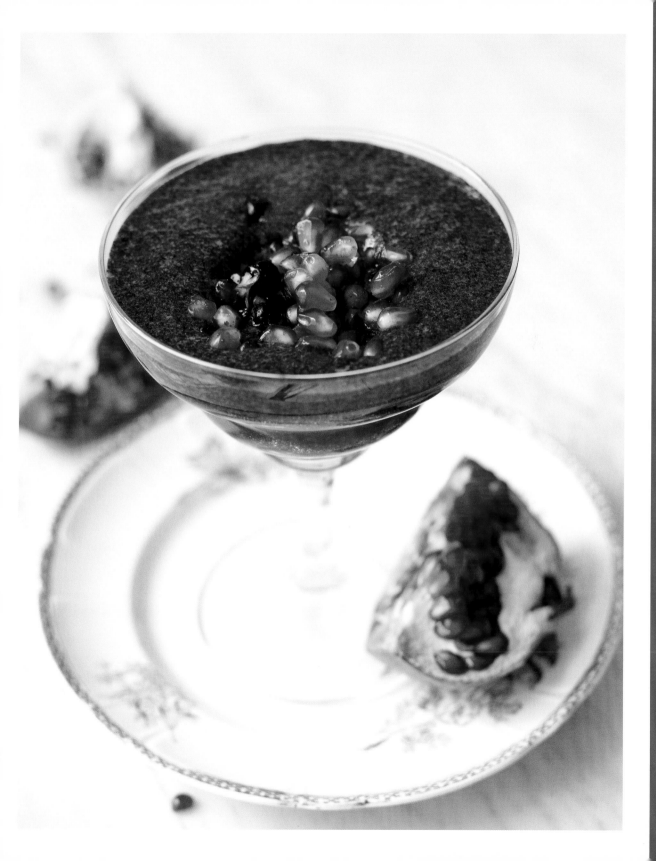

Breakfast Juices

Introduce a new habit and kickstart your morning with cleansing juices made from vegetables, herbs, and fruits!

WAKE ME UP GREEN DRINK

135 CALORIES/SERVES 2

½ pineapple
1 fennel bulb
½ hothouse cucumber
Juice from 1 lime
1 large bunch Italian parsley
2½ cups (6 dl) water

1. Peel the pineapple and cut away the hard core in the middle. Cut the fruit into pieces. Cut away the bottom part of the fennel bulb and the middle core. Slice the rest. Cut the cucumber into big pieces. Put everything in a blender.
2. Add the lime juice, parsley leaves, and water. Blend to a smooth mixture and pour into a glass or a pitcher.

DETOX MY MORNING

75 CALORIES/SERVES 2

2 tablespoons fresh grated ginger
Juice of 1½ lemons
1½ tablespoons agave syrup
1 teaspoon cayenne pepper
2½ cups (6 dl) water

1. Mix all ingredients in a pitcher. Serve in a glass or pour into a bottle.

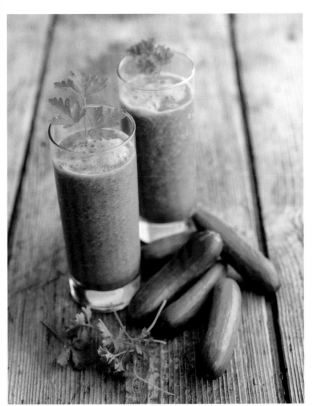

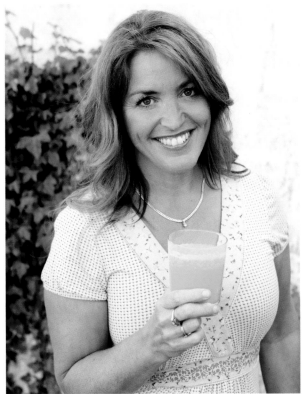

> *Cayenne pepper is excellent for stoking your metabolism.*

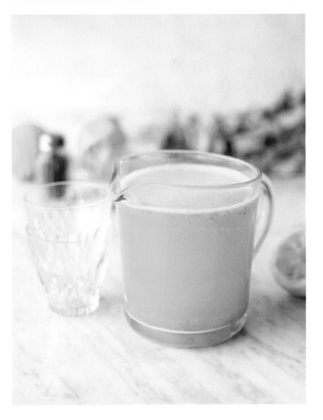

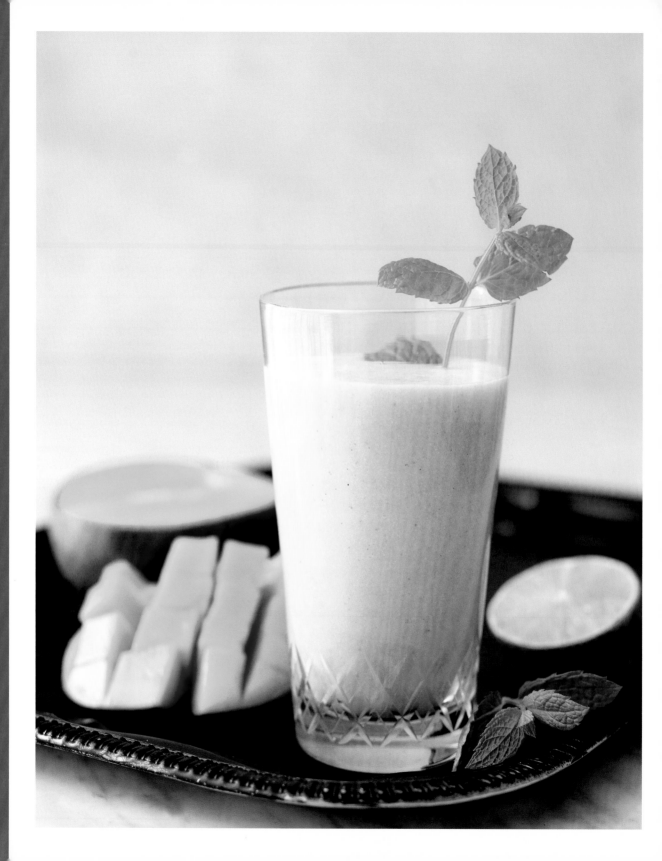

YELLOW SUNSHINE
Smoothie

*Absolutely delicious smoothie full of wonderful flavors.
It is also full of nutrients and makes you feel full—that can't be bad, can it?*

481 CALORIES/SERVES 2

1 orange
7 ounces (200 g) diced
   mango, frozen
14 ounces (400 g)
   coconut milk
1 tablespoon agave
   syrup
2 teaspoons fresh
   grated ginger
½ teaspoon vanilla
   powder
1¼ cup (3 dl) water
Juice from 1 lime
Fresh mint as desired +
   some for garnish

1. Peel the orange and cut it into pieces. Place the pieces in a blender along with the remaining ingredients and blend to make a smoothie.
2. Pour into a glass and garnish with a sprig of mint—or pour into a bottle.

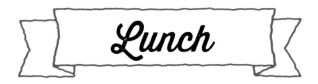

ENERGY DRINK

A cleansing smoothie with lemon and ginger. Try variations using other fruits such as kiwi, mango, and banana instead of pineapple. Store the pitcher in the refrigerator and drink a glass now and then, or take it with you in a bottle.

367 CALORIES/SERVES 1

1 lemon
6¾ ounces (2 dl)
  spinach leaves
1 bunch parsley
1 hothouse cucumber
1 stalk celery
1 avocado
6¾ ounces (2 dl) diced
  frozen pineapple
1 tablespoon fresh
  grated ginger
1¾ cups (3 dl) water

1. Peel the lemon with a sharp knife and dice the lemon. Put in a blender together with spinach and parsley (sprigs and leaves).
2. Slice the cucumber, celery, and avocado flesh and place all of it in the blender together with pineapple, ginger, and water.
3. Blend to make a smoothie and pour into a pitcher or a bottle.

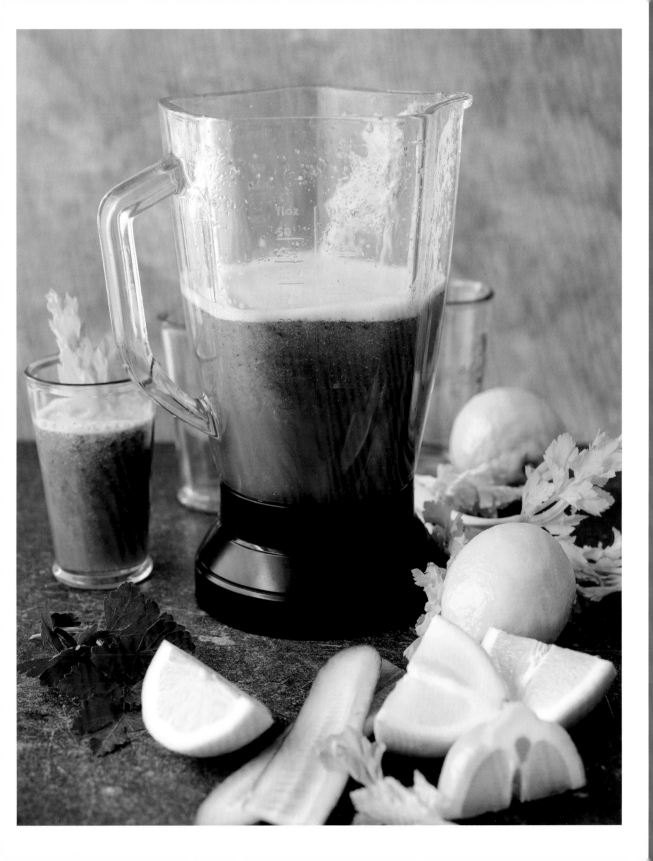

RED DELICIOUS
Lunch Drink

A juice with vitamins A, C, and K, iron, and folic acid! Beets strengthen the liver and have cleansing properties. The chia seeds fill you up and provide antioxidants and omega-3 fatty acids.

135 CALORIES/SERVES 2

2 fresh beets
½ hothouse cucumber
1 stalk celery
2½ cups (6 dl) water
Juice from 1 lemon
2 tablespoons chia seeds

1. Peel and slice the beets and put them in a blender. Cut the cucumber and celery into smaller pieces. Add them to the blender and mix it all to an even mixture. Add the water and lemon juice and blend some more. Pour into a glass or pitcher and then stir in the chia seeds.
2. Let sit at least 20 minutes before serving.

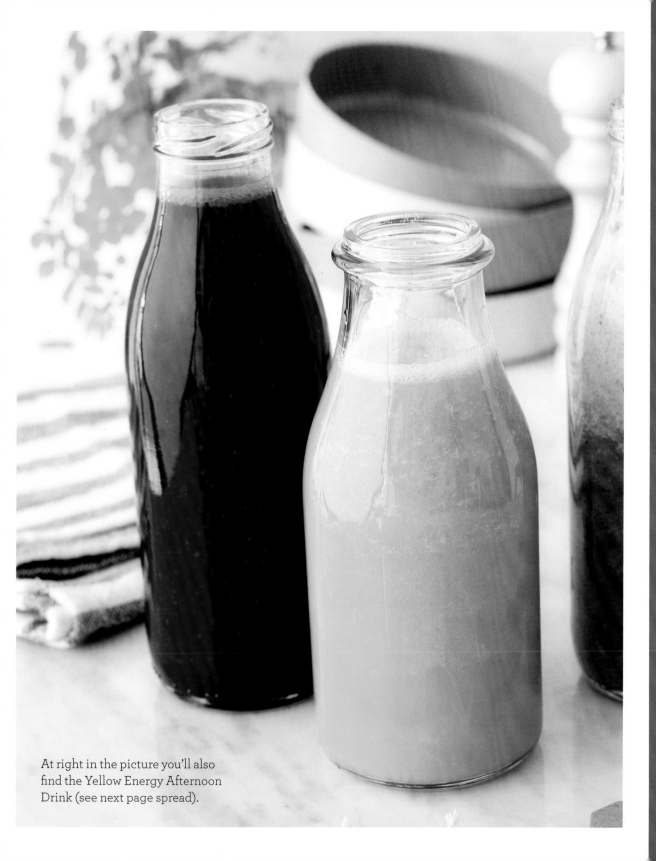

At right in the picture you'll also find the Yellow Energy Afternoon Drink (see next page spread).

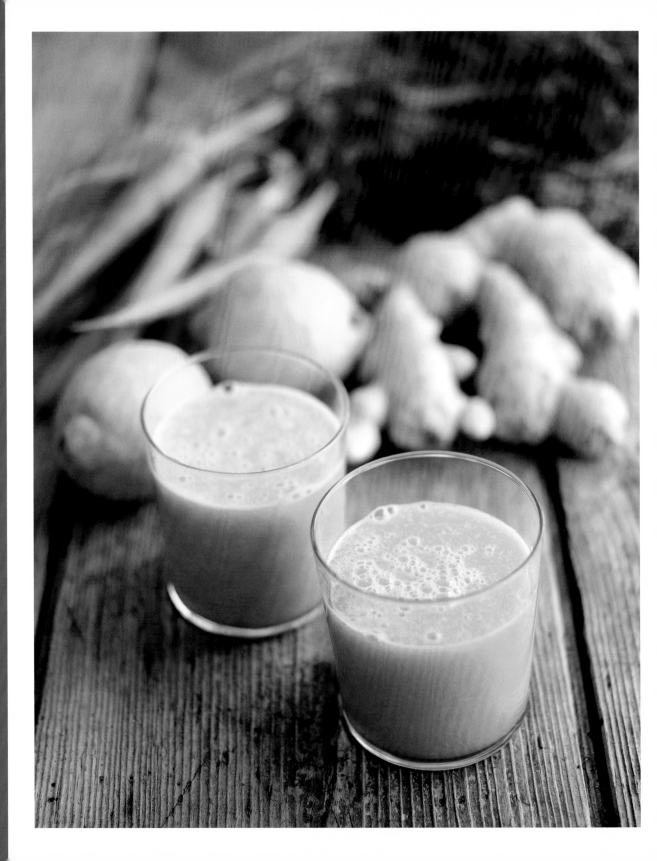

YELLOW ENERGY
Afternoon Drink

A slightly tart juice with plenty of the cleansing ginger root.
The juice will keep your blood glucose level as it simultaneously
provides an energy boost. The turmeric is an anti-inflammatory.

160 CALORIES/SERVES 2

2 carrots
1 red apple
1 orange
½ teaspoon turmeric
Juice of 1 lemon
**1 tablespoon fresh
  grated ginger**
3 cups (7 dl) water

1. Cut the carrots and apple into smaller pieces.
   Peel the orange and cut it into pieces.
2. Place all the ingredients in a blender and mix to
   make a smoothie.
3. Pour into a glass or a pitcher.

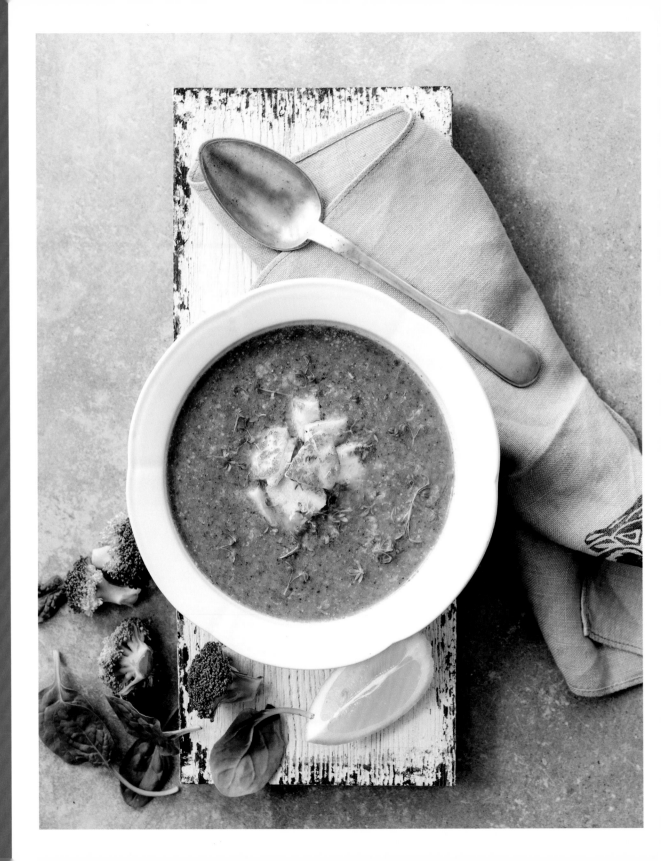

Broccoli and Spinach Soup
WITH HALLOUMI

Filling soup full of iron, vitamin K, and chlorophyll!

285 CALORIES/SERVES 4

1 yellow onion
1 clove garlic
1 teaspoon olive oil
3 cups (7 dl) water
2 tablespoons organic, gluten-free stock powder
1 stalk broccoli with florets
7 ounces (200 g) fresh spinach
7 ounces (200 g) coconut cream
Salt
Black pepper

Topping

5¼ ounces (150 g) halloumi
1 teaspoon olive oil
Some water cress
Grated lemon peel

1. Chop the onion and garlic. Heat the oil in a large saucepan and fry the onion and garlic. Add the water and stock powder and bring to a boil.
2. Cut the broccoli into pieces and place in the saucepan along with the spinach leaves. Let simmer over low heat for about 10 minutes.
3. Blend the soup until smooth and add in the coconut cream. Season with salt and pepper.
4. Cut the halloumi into pieces and fry in oil until they are nicely colored.
5. Divide the soup between bowls and top with halloumi, cress, and grated lemon peel.

BLOODY MARY
Cleansing Beauty

A juice with some heat that also provides satiety. The ginger root and cayenne pepper give the metabolism a kick!

73 CALORIES/SERVES 2

½ **quart (½ liter) tomato juice**
Juice from ½ lemon
Juice from ½ lime
2 **teaspoons fresh grated ginger**
⅕ **teaspoon (1 krm) cayenne pepper**
Salt
Black pepper
2 **celery stalks, for garnish**

1. Pour the tomato juice into a pitcher and add the rest of the ingredients except celery.
2. Mix thoroughly and pour into a glass or a bottle. Serve garnished with a celery stalk.

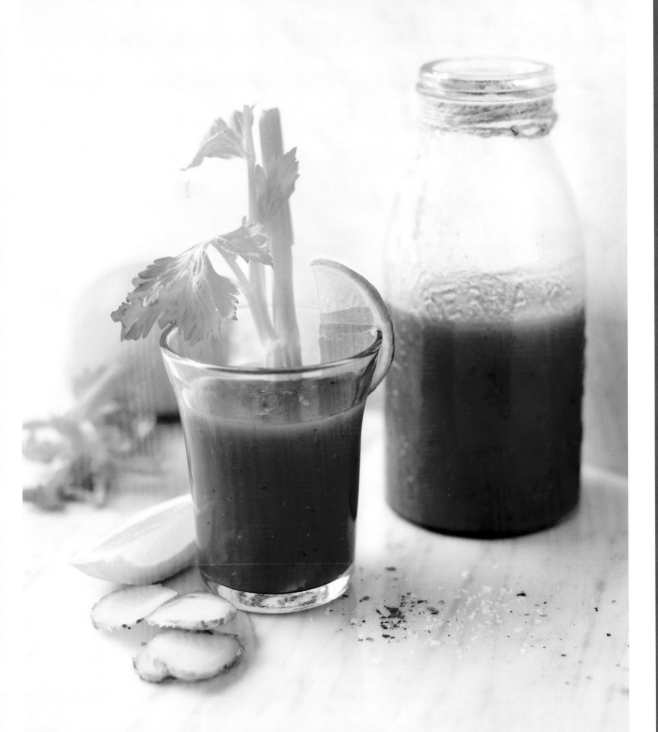

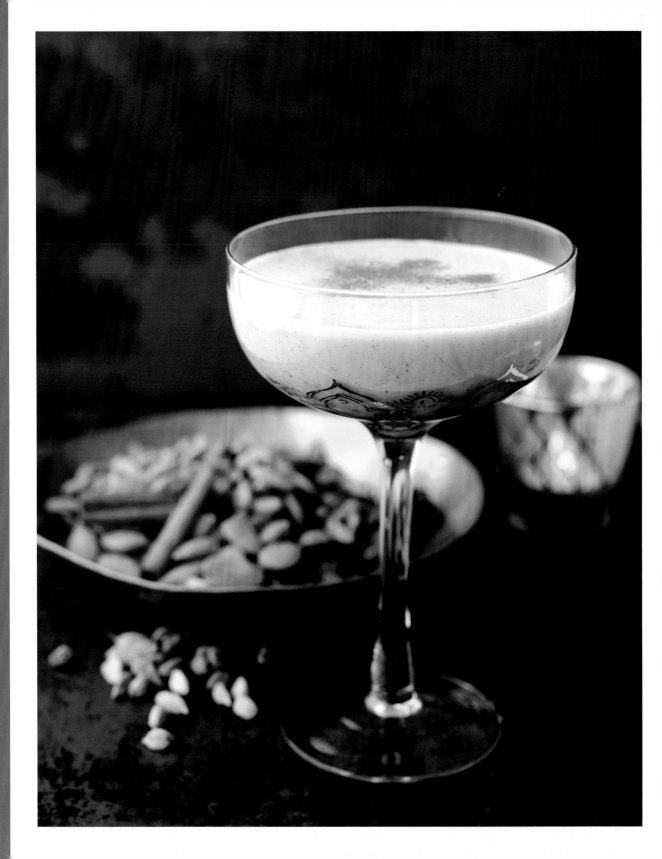

GOOD NIGHT
Milky Drink

Almond milk is rich in protein and vitamins D and E. They strengthen skin, hair, and nails. This is a beverage to look forward to, since it helps you get a good night's sleep.

153 CALORIES/SERVES 2

5 dried pitted dates
⅕ teaspoon (1 krm) salt
1½ teaspoons ground cinnamon
1½ teaspoons ground cardamom
½ teaspoon vanilla powder
3 cups (7 dl) almond milk
Cinnamon for sprinkling, optional

1. Quickly blend the dates and spices in a mixer. Add the almond milk a bit at a time while continuing to blend.
2. Pour into a glass and sprinkle with some ground cinnamon, if desired. Can also be bottled.

FIFTY SHADES OF
Green Drink

A green drink that will fill you up nicely. Here you have a mix of many good things such as broccoli, which provides vitamin C, calcium, iron, and Vitamin K.

280 CALORIES/SERVES 2

1 avocado

2 kiwifruit + slices for garnish

1½ oranges

½ banana

½ hothouse cucumber

5 broccoli florets

A few pea shoots + extra for garnish

Juice of 1 lime

1¾ cups (4 dl) almond milk

6¾ fluid ounces (2 dl) water

1. Peel the avocado and remove the pit. Peel the kiwifruit, orange, and banana and place everything in a blender. Quickly blend.

2. Cut the cucumber and broccoli into smaller pieces and place them in the blender with the pea shoots.

3. Add the lime juice, almond milk, and water. Blend to a smooth mixture and pour into a glass. Garnish with kiwifruit slices and pea shoots.

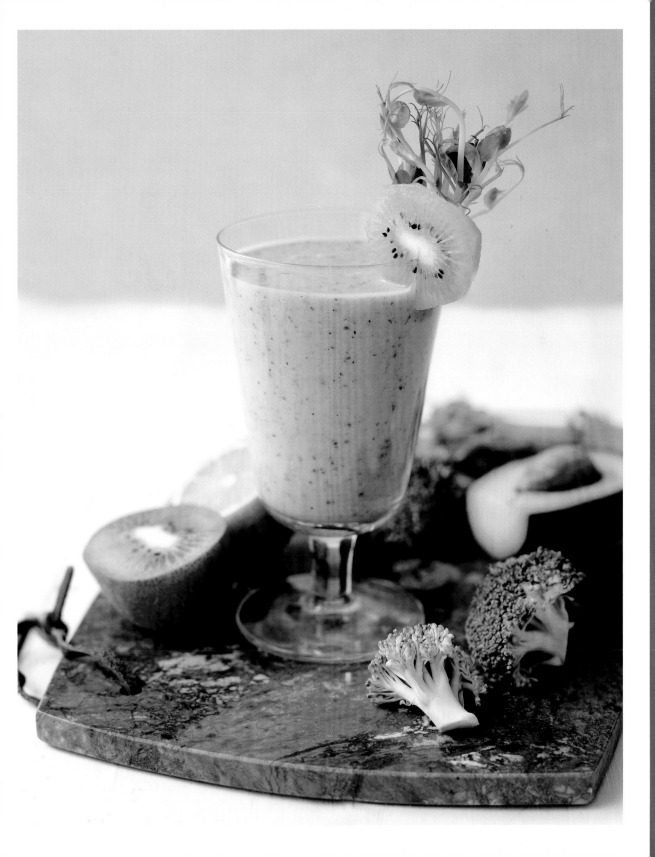

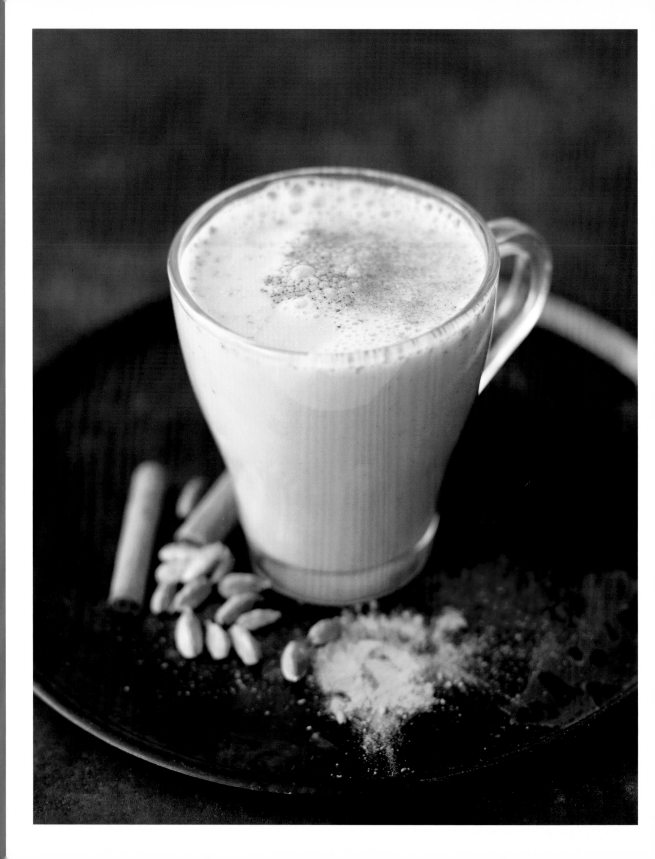

Golden
NIGHTCAP MILK

A tasty and warming nightcap. It is cleansing and anti-inflammatory and can provide relief from joint pain.

104 CALORIES/SERVES 1

1 teaspoon turmeric paste
1¼ cups (3 dl) oat or almond milk
½ teaspoon ground cardamom
½ teaspoon vanilla powder
Pinch cayenne pepper
Pinch black pepper
½ teaspoon honey
Some grated fresh ginger
Ground cinnamon for sprinkling

1. Warm the turmeric paste and milk in a saucepan, and stir in the rest of the ingredients except cinnamon.
2. Pour into a cup or glass. Sprinkle with some ground cinnamon.

TURMERIC PASTE

1¾ ounces (½ dl) organic ground turmeric
5 ounces (1½ dl) water
Black pepper

1. Mix the ingredients in a saucepan and bring to a boil while stirring. Lower the heat and keep stirring a while longer.
2. Add more water if the paste becomes too thick.
3. Store the turmeric paste in the refrigerator. It will keep for several weeks and is enough for many servings.

Asian Cauliflower Soup

A feast both for the eyes and the palate!
I constantly come back to this recipe.

476 CALORIES/SERVES 2

½ small cauliflower
2 carrots
1 salad onion
1 small clove garlic
1 tablespoon olive oil
1 tablespoon fresh grated ginger
Salt
Black pepper
Approximately 1¼ cups (3 dl) water
1 vegetarian or organic gluten-free stock cube
1 small can (6 fluid ounces/165 ml) coconut milk
1–2 tablespoons red Thai curry paste
1 teaspoon honey
Juice from ½ lime

Topping

Fried cauliflower florets
4 tablespoons salted peanuts, coarsely chopped
2 tablespoons salad onion, julienned
Fresh cilantro
Julienned chili pepper

1. Cut the cauliflower, carrots, and salad onion into smaller pieces. Finely chop the garlic. Heat the oil in a saucepan and fry it all together with the ginger for about a minute. Season with salt and pepper.
2. Add the water, crumbled stock cube, coconut milk, curry paste, honey, and lime juice. Let simmer for about 10 minutes.
3. With an immersion blender or in a food processor, mix the soup until smooth. Dilute with more water if needed. Taste the soup and add more curry paste, spices, or lime juice as needed.
4. Pour the soup into bowls and sprinkle with the toppings.

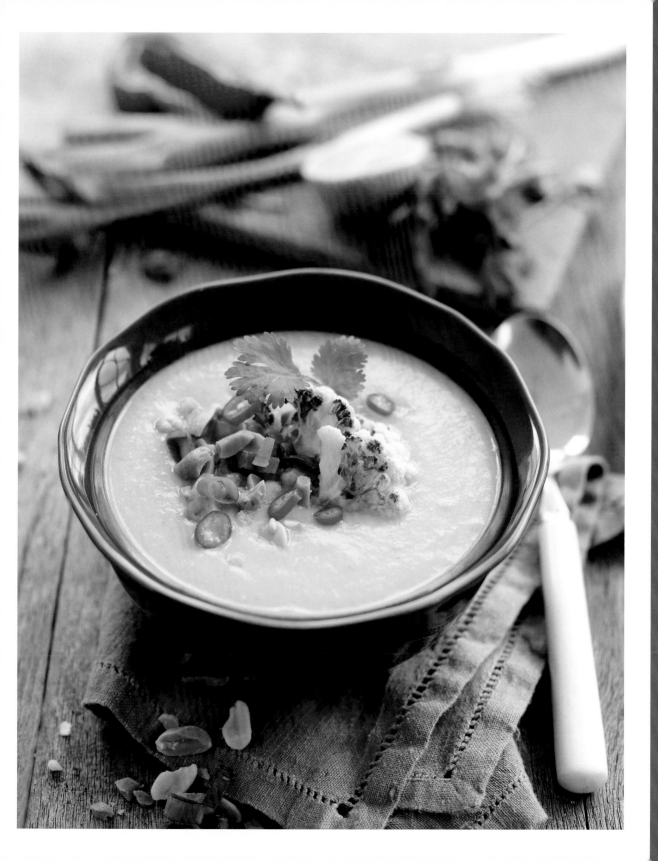

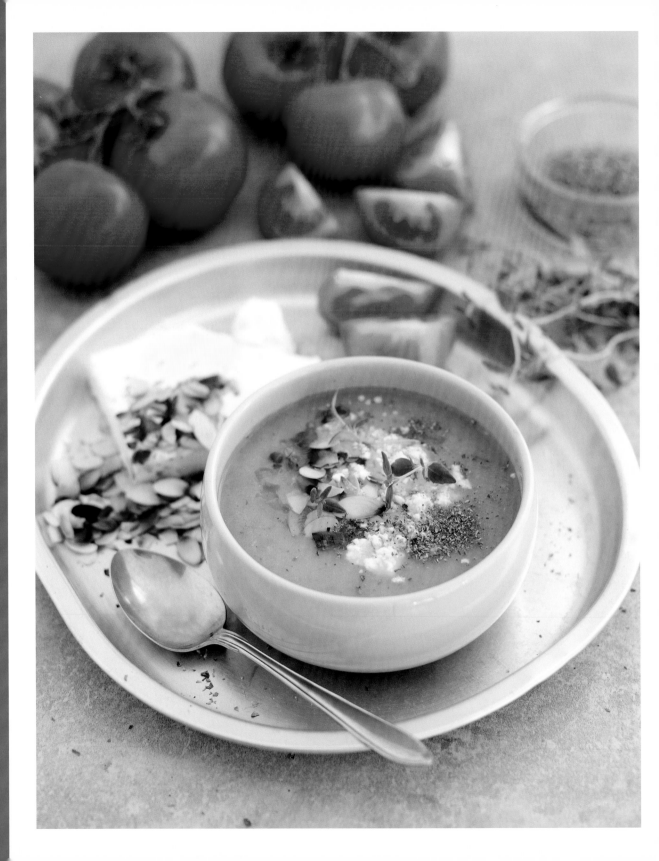

Tomato and Carrot Soup
WITH FETA CHEESE AND SLIVERED ALMONDS

A filling and easy-to-prepare tomato soup, with a topping that enhances all good flavors.

290 CALORIES/SERVES 4

6 medium tomatoes, still on the vine
1 large yellow onion
2 carrots
½ red chili
4 dried pitted dates
1 tablespoon olive oil
1 clove garlic, pressed
2½ cups (6 dl) water
1 teaspoon honey
2 teaspoons organic, gluten-free stock powder
1 teaspoon dried Mediterranean oregano
Salt
Black pepper

Topping

1¾ ounces (50 g) slivered almonds
5¼ ounces (150 g) feta cheese
Fresh thyme
Dried Mediterranean oregano

1. Cut the tomatoes into smaller pieces. Chop the onion and coarsely grate the carrots. Finely chop the chili and chop the dates.
2. Heat the oil in a saucepan and fry all the vegetables for a few minutes. Add the dates, garlic, water, honey, stock powder, and spices. Bring the soup to a boil and let it simmer for 5 minutes.
3. With an immersion blender, mix the soup until smooth and pour it back into the saucepan and reheat it. Season with salt and pepper.
4. Roast the almond slivers in a dry skillet while stirring. Pour the soup into deep bowls and top with crumbled feta cheese. Top with slivered almonds, thyme, and oregano.

Lentil Soup
WITH HALLOUMI

*A flavorful, beautiful, and filling soup. Carrots, cinnamon,
and coconut milk round out the flavors wonderfully.*

517 CALORIES/SERVES 2

½ yellow onion
1 clove garlic
1 carrot
1 tablespoon canola oil
1 tablespoon fresh grated
   ginger
½ tablespoon curry
1 vegetable stock cube
Approximately 1¾ cups
   (4 dl) water
6¾ fluid ounces (2 dl)
   coconut milk
1 tablespoon sweet chili
   sauce or 1 teaspoon
   sambal oelek
A heaped 5 fluid ounces
   (1½ dl) red lentils
1 cinnamon stick
Salt
Black pepper

Topping

3½ ounces (100 g)
   halloumi
Fine strips of leek
Fine strips of red onion
Some chervil leaves

1. Chop the onion and garlic. Peel and slice the
   carrot. Heat the oil in a saucepan and fry the
   onion, garlic, carrot, ginger, and curry for a
   minute. Crumble in the stock cube and add the
   water, coconut milk, and sweet chili sauce. Stir
   in the lentils and add the cinnamon stick.

2. Let cook over low heat for about 15 minutes.
   Dilute with more water if needed. Season with
   salt and pepper. Remove the cinnamon stick and
   blend the soup until smooth. Pour the soup into
   bowls.

3. Dice the halloumi and fry it in some oil. Top
   the soup with the dice and leek, red onion, and
   chervil.

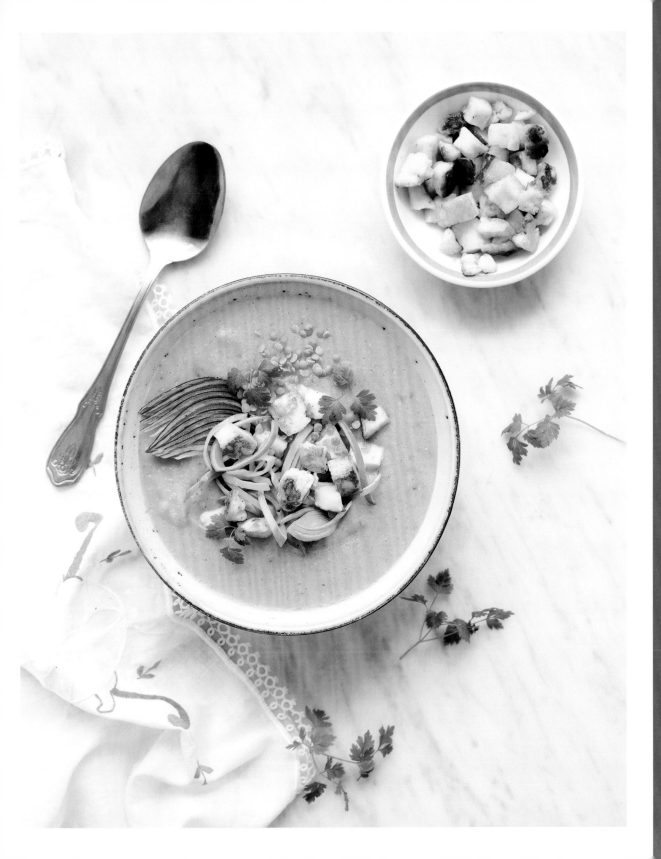

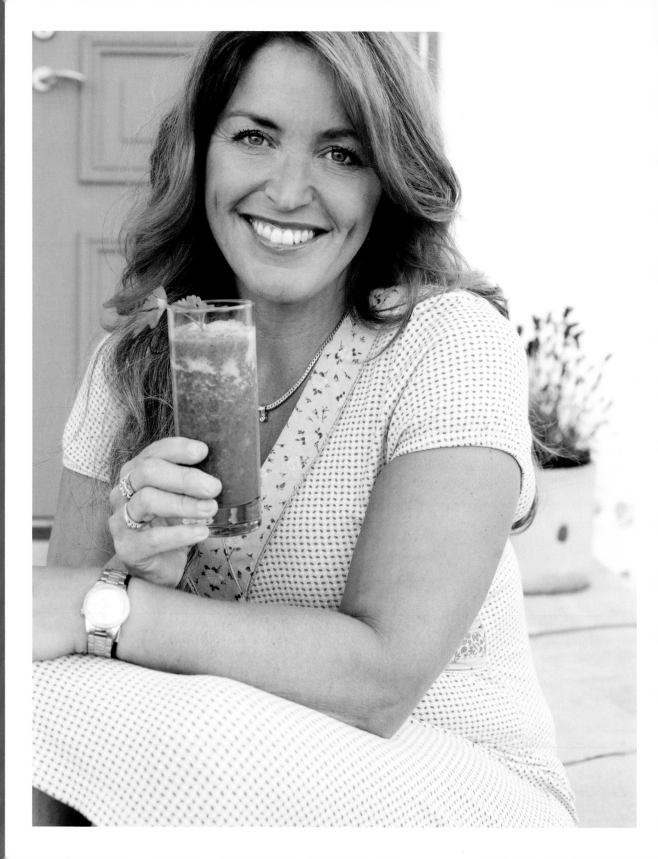

JUICING
Meal Schedule

DURATION: 1 WEEK
WEIGHT LOSS: 6½ TO 8¾ POUNDS (3–4 KG)

Welcome to a world full of colorful juices! In this kickstart you start by scaling down for one day—this means giving up sugar, gluten, dairy products, animal protein, alcohol and coffee. Then follow four days of juice fasting, when you drink six extremely nutritious juices each day between 8 a.m. and 8 p.m. The interval between drinks is between two and three hours.

You'll finish your juice fast with two days of ramping up with delicious smoothies and soups. Make sure to drink plenty of lemon water, preferably lukewarm (see recipe on p. 143) during the week.

You'll take in quite few calories over those days—between 730 and 1,600—but the calories you do consume will be nourishing, filling, and full of fiber.

As the juices contain primarily vegetables, and the quantity of fruit is small, your blood glucose will stay level. If you get hungry between drinks, fill up on lemon water and enjoy tasty herb teas or a miso soup.

This meal schedule lasts one week, which can be just the right amount for a first timer.

DAY	BREAKFAST	LUNCH	DINNER
Monday **1,264 calories**	Red Blueberry Dream Smoothie, p. 148 (322 calories)	Broccoli and Spinach Soup with Halloumi, p. 161 (285 calories)—freeze at least one serving! 1 pitcher Green Energy Drink, p. 154 (367 calories)	Tomato and Carrot Soup with Feta Cheese and Slivered Almonds, p. 173 (290 calories)—freeze at least one serving!
Tuesday **731 calories**	8 A.M.—Detox My Morning, p. 150 (75 calories) 10 A.M.—Wake Me Up Green Drink, p. 150 (135 calories)	12 P.M.—Red Delicious Lunch Drink, p. 156 (135 calories) 3 P.M.—Yellow Energy Afternoon Drink, p. 159 (160 calories)	6 P.M.—Bloody Mary Cleansing Beauty, p. 162 (73 calories) 8 P.M.—Good Night Milky Drink, p. 165 (153 calories)
Wednesday **731 calories**	8 A.M.—Detox My Morning, p. 150 (75 calories) 10 A.M.—Wake Me Up Green Drink, p. 150 (135 calories)	12 P.M.—Red Delicious Lunch Drink, p. 156 (135 calories) 3 P.M.—Yellow Energy Afternoon Drink, p. 159 (160 calories)	6 P.M.—Bloody Mary Cleansing Beauty, p. 162 (73 calories) 8 P.M.—Good Night Milky Drink, p. 165 (153 calories)
Thursday **967 calories**	8 A.M.—3 servings Slim-Down Raspberry Drink, p. 112 (153 calories total) 10 A.M.—Wake Me Up Green Drink, p. 150 (135 calories)	12 P.M.—Red Delicious Lunch Drink, p. 156 (135 calories) 3 P.M.—Yellow Afternoon Energy Drink, p. 159 (160 calories)	6 P.M.—Fifty Shades of Green Drink, p. 166 (280 calories) 8 P.M.—Golden Nightcap Milk, p. 169 (104 calories)
Friday **967 calories**	8 A.M.—3 servings Slim-Down Raspberry Drink, p. 112 (153 calories total) 10 A.M.—Wake Me Up Green Drink, p. 150 (135 calories)	12 P.M.—Red Delicious Lunch Drink, p. 156 (135 calories) 3 P.M.—Yellow Afternoon Energy Drink, p. 159 (160 calories)	6 P.M.—Fifty Shades of Green Drink, p. 166 (280 calories) 8 P.M.—Golden Nightcap Milk, p. 169 (104 calories)
Saturday **1,588 calories**	Red Blueberry Dream Smoothie, p. 148 (322 calories)	Tomato and Carrot Soup with Feta Cheese and Slivered Almonds (290 calories), *leftovers*	Asian Cauliflower Soup, p. 170 (476 calories) Melon Boats, p. 182 (500 calories)
Sunday **1,283 calories**	Yellow Sunshine Smoothie, p. 153 (481 calories)	Broccoli and Spinach Soup with Halloumi (285 calories), *leftovers*	Lentil Soup with Halloumi, p. 170 (517 calories)

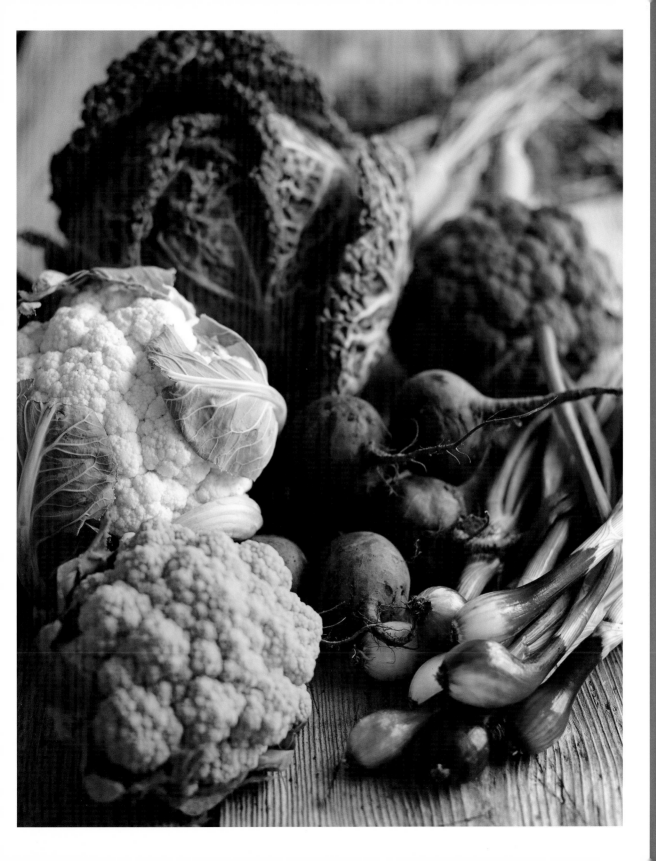

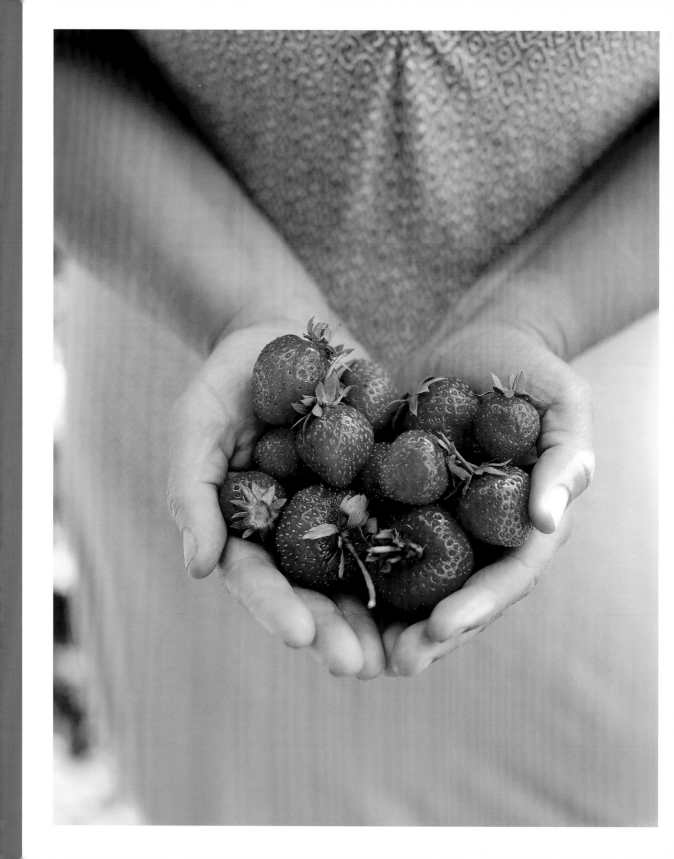

DESSERTS & SNACKS

Life must have balance and be enjoyable! Here I'll offer you good-for-you desserts and snacks that have a lot of fruit, berries, nuts, and pure, raw ingredients. The recipes are free of refined sugar, gluten, and cow's milk, without losing their deliciousness. Quite the opposite, in fact! You are really going to enjoy these treats. Best of all, you can do it with a clean conscience!

Below is some information about the ingredients in this chapter:

Almond flour can be found in the health food section or among the baking products. It is gluten-free and is suitable for baking.

Soy yogurt is in the dairy section in most grocery stores. Preferably choose a plain variety.

Tofutti cream cheese is a dairy-free alternative to crème fraîche and is both tasty and useful in vegetarian and vegan foods, and also in baked goods. It will be in the dairy section in well-stocked grocery stores.

Coconut milk and coconut cream are the perfect alternatives to dairy milk and cream.

Honey has the same energy content as common table sugar but is more natural and contains some vitamins and minerals. Nice in baked goods, on yogurt, and in tea. Try to find organic, local honey!

Agave syrup is extracted from a cactus and causes minimal rise in blood glucose. Contains a smidgen more fructose than glucose, and should be used with caution, because the liver is the only organ that can break down any excess fructose. Excellent flavor carrier in desserts, baked goods, and savory dishes, and also very easy to measure.

Vanilla powder is the ground vanilla bean without any additives; it has a naturally sweet flavor. Use this instead of vanilla sugar. Try to find the organic variety.

Melon Boats

Simple and fresh luxury: cut a melon or pineapple in half and scoop out the inside. Fill the halves with mixed fruits and berries. Delicious!

500 CALORIES/SERVES 2

1 Santa Claus melon, honeydew melon, or pineapple
2 oranges
1 red apple
1 mango

Marinade

Juice of 1 lime
1 passion fruit
2 tablespoons honey or other sweetener
½ bunch of mint, chopped

Topping

½ passion fruit
2 lime slices
2 tablespoons coconut flakes
Fresh raspberries

1. Halve the melon lengthwise and remove the seeds and the contents of the fruit. Cut the melon into pieces and place in a bowl. Dice the oranges, apple, and mango and add to the bowl.
2. Mix all ingredients for the marinade in a bowl. Stir until the honey has dissolved. Stir the marinade into the bowl with the fruit and mix thoroughly.
3. Serve the fruit salad in the scooped-out melon halves and top with passion fruit, lime slices, coconut flakes, and raspberries.

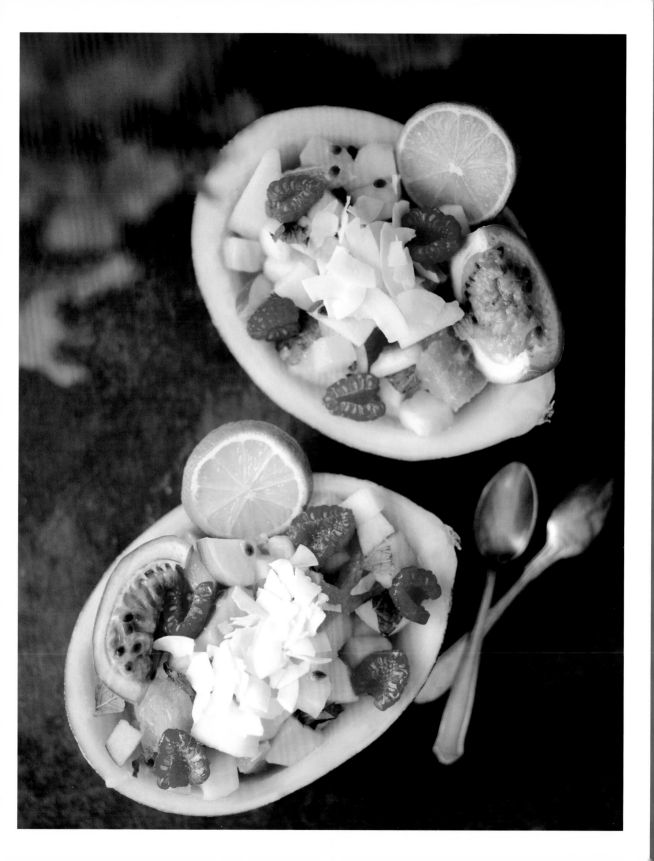

Sorbet and Ice Cream

Enjoy a refreshing sorbet made with your favorite berries. Summer flavors year-round! Or why not a creamy ice cream with a spike of mint flavor?

BERRY SORBET

75 CALORIES/SERVES 4

1 pound frozen mixed berries (for example blackberries, blueberries, raspberries, and strawberries)
1 pound plain soy yogurt
½ teaspoon vanilla powder
1 tablespoon honey

To serve
6¾ ounces (2 dl) fresh or frozen berries

1. Place all the ingredients in a food processor and process to a smooth mixture. Spread the mixture evenly in a pan and cover it with plastic wrap and leave it in the freezer for at least 4 hours.
2. Remove the pan from the freezer about 20 minutes before serving. Scoop the sorbet into bowls and serve with berries.

MANGO AND COCONUT ICE CREAM WITH MINT

129 CALORIES/SERVES 4

1 pound frozen diced mango
7 ounces (200 g) coconut cream
1¾ ounces (½ dl) fresh mint leaves + extra for garnish

1. Place all the ingredients in a food processor and process to a smooth mixture. Spread the mixture evenly in a pan and cover it with plastic wrap. Leave it in the freezer for at least 4 hours.
2. Remove the ice cream from the freezer about 20 minutes before serving. Scoop the ice cream into bowls and garnish with mint.

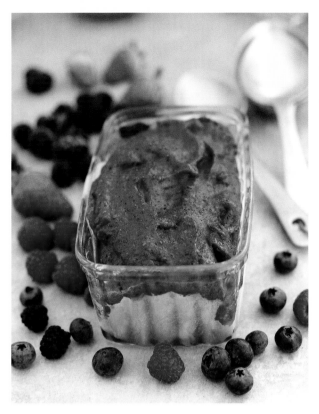

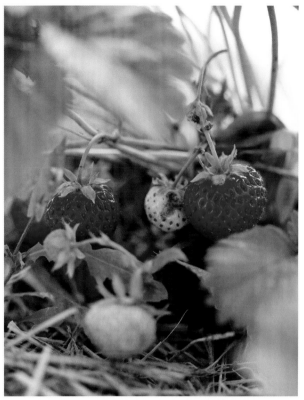

Place ice cream and sorbet at room temperature for 20 minutes before serving— that way they will be easier to scoop.

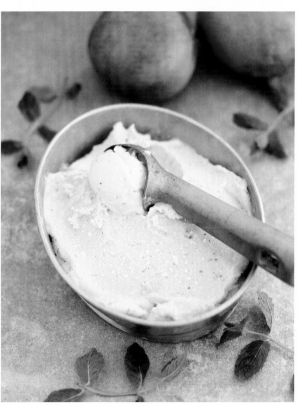

Chocolate Crisp
WITH QUINOA

Absolutely wonderful chocolate squares! Bake and enjoy with friends or colleagues—these small treats will disappear quickly.

APPROXIMATELY 165 CALORIES/MAKES ABOUT 20 PIECES

2 tablespoons coconut oil

1½ tablespoons agave syrup

⅕ teaspoon (1 krm) vanilla powder

3⅓ ounces (1 dl) white quinoa

3⅓ ounces (1 dl) pumpkin seeds, chopped

1¾ ounces (½ dl) sunflower seeds

1¾ ounces (½ dl) pecans, chopped

2 teaspoons chia seed

2 teaspoons hemp hearts

Topping

7 ounces (200 g) dark chocolate, about 70% cacao

2 tablespoons hemp hearts for sprinkling

1. Preheat the oven to 400°F (200°C). Melt the coconut oil in a saucepan and then pour it into a bowl along with the agave syrup and vanilla powder. Add the remaining ingredients and mix thoroughly.

2. Spread the batter on a baking sheet lined with parchment paper. Place another piece of parchment paper on top and use it to spread the batter out into a thin, flat cake. Remove the top paper and bake the cake in the middle of the oven for 20 minutes. Let it cool completely.

3. Melt the chocolate over a double-boiler. and spread it evenly over the cake. Sprinkle with hemp hearts and let the cake set in the refrigerator for 30 minutes. Break the cake into approximately 20 pieces and store them in the refrigerator.

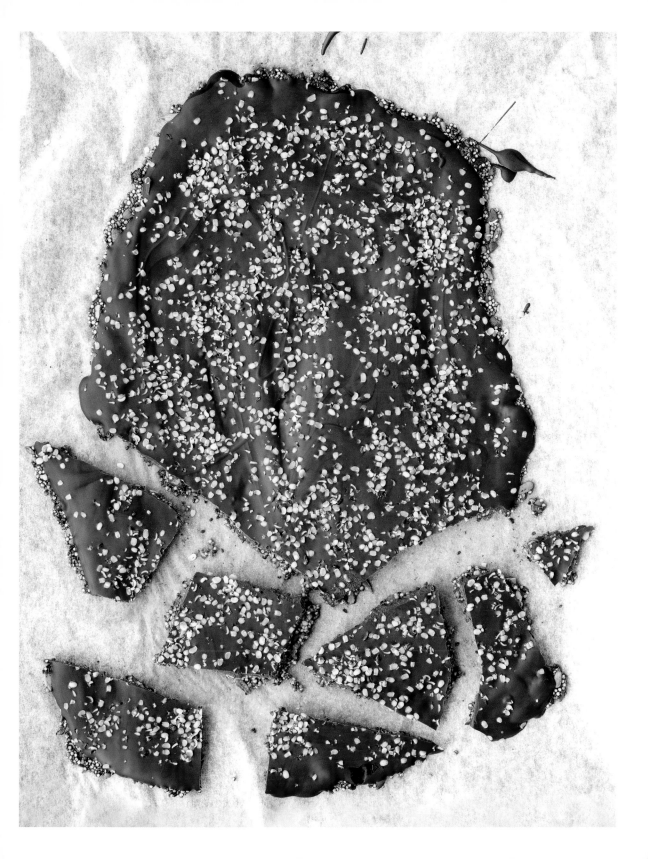

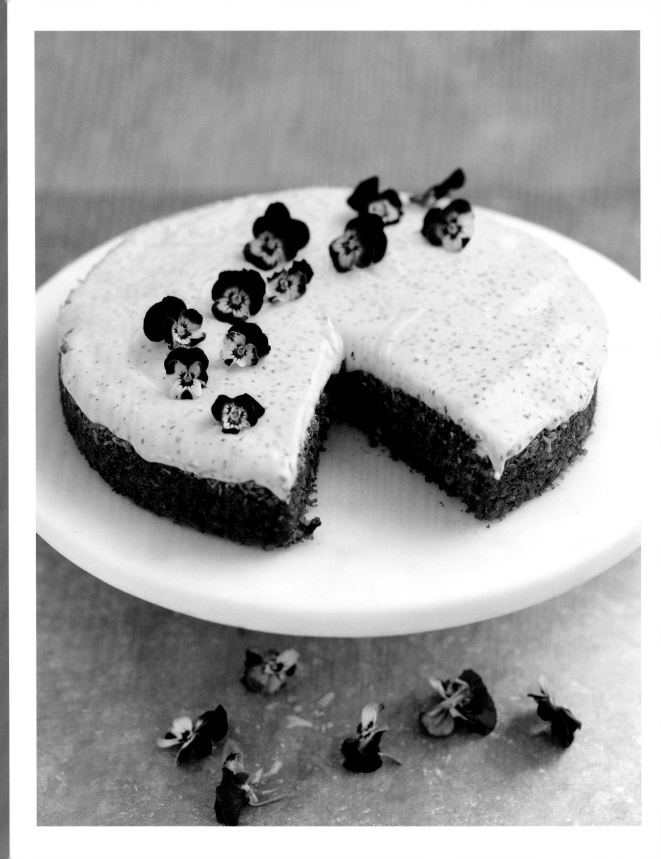

Beet Cake
WITH SAFFRON CRÈME

This cake's flavor and texture will be even better if you bake it a day ahead.
You can replace Tofutti cream cheese with your preferred brand.

535 CALORIES/SERVING. – **SERVES 8**

1 teaspoon sunflower oil + ⅓ cup (¾ dl) coconut flakes for the baking pan

1¾ cups (4 dl) almond flour

½ teaspoon salt

2 teaspoons ground cardamom

1 tablespoon ground cinnamon

½ teaspoon ground nutmeg

1 teaspoon baking soda

⅕ teaspoon (1 krm) vanilla powder

1½ cups (3½ dl) sunflower oil

3 eggs

3⅓ fluid ounces (1 dl) agave syrup

1¾ cup (4 dl) raw beets, grated

1¼ cups (3 dl) walnuts, chopped

Saffron crème

½ pound (225 g) Tofutti cream cheese

2 tablespoons agave syrup

1-portion envelope saffron (½ g)

Garnish

Edible flowers or spiralized fresh beets

1. Preheat the oven to 350°F (175°C). Oil a springform pan about 9½ inches (24 cm) in diameter and cover the inside with coconut flakes.
2. Mix the dry cake ingredients in a bowl. Add the oil and eggs and whisk to a smooth batter. Add the syrup, beets, and walnuts and mix thoroughly. Pour the batter into the springform pan and bake in the middle of the oven for 40 minutes. Let the cake cool completely.
3. Mix cream cheese, syrup, and saffron and spread the frosting over the cake. Garnish with flowers or something else that looks pretty.

Raw Mango Cake

You'll need to plan ahead for this cake since both buckwheat and cashews require soaking. However, you can freeze these ingredients if you have soaked them properly. They'll defrost in 20 minutes.

441 CALORIES/SERVES 8

Bottom layer

3⅓ ounces (1 dl) whole buckwheat
6¾ ounces (2 dl) walnuts
10 dried pitted dates
2 tablespoons agave syrup

Mango crème

1¾ cups (4 dl) plain cashews
2 mangoes
½ teaspoon turmeric
4 tablespoons agave syrup
2 tablespoons coconut oil

Topping

1 mango, diced
3½ ounces (100 g) fresh blueberries
1 tablespoon freeze-dried blueberries

1. Rinse the buckwheat in boiling water (see explanation on how to do this on p. 88). Leave it to soak in cold water for 8 hours or overnight. Let the cashews for the mango crème soak in water for 8 hours or overnight, too, but in a separate bowl.

2. Drain the buckwheat and cashews and rinse thoroughly (and separately) with cold water. Let them dry out a little.

3. Place the buckwheat, walnuts, dates, and agave syrup in a food processor and process to a coarse batter. Press out the batter into a 9½-inch (24 cm) diameter springform pan and leave it in the freezer until the mango crème is made.

4. Cut the mango into pieces and place in a food processor together with the remaining mango crème ingredients. Process until you have a smooth mixture. Remove the cake from the freezer and spread the mixture evenly on top. Return the cake to the freezer for at least 3 hours.

5. Remove the cake from the freezer about 15 minutes before serving, and garnish it with fresh mango pieces, blueberries, and freeze-dried blueberries.

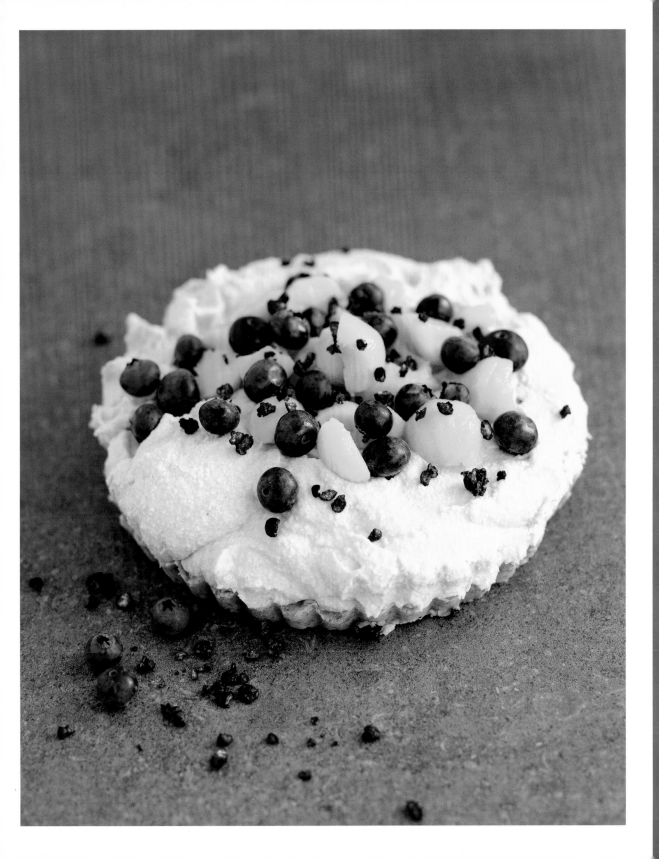

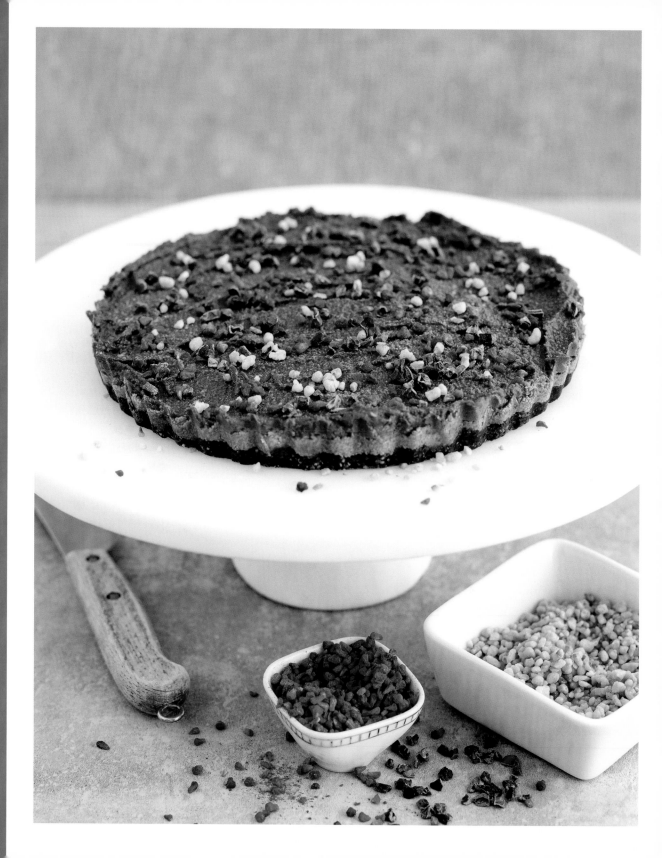

Raw Raspberry
AND CHOCOLATE CAKE

The best cake, made without sugar and gluten flour! Perfect for storing in the freezer and bringing out for a coffee break or for dessert.

303 CALORIES/SERVES 8

Bottom layer

3⅓ ounces (1 dl) almonds

3½ ounces (1 dl) dried pitted dates

1½ tablespoons cocoa

¼ teaspoon vanilla powder

1¾ ounces (50 gr) dark chocolate, 70% cacao

1 teaspoon coconut oil

Raspberry filling

3⅓ ounces frozen raspberries

1¾ ounces (½ dl) raw cashews

2 tablespoons coconut flakes

3 tablespoons agave syrup

½ teaspoon fresh lemon juice

4 tablespoons melted coconut oil

Chocolate filling

3⅓ ounces (1 dl) raw cashews

2 tablespoons coconut oil

1 tablespoon cocoa

2 tablespoons agave syrup

Topping

Freeze-dried raspberries

Chopped hazelnuts/filberts

Cacao nibs

1. In a food processor, mix the almonds, dates, cocoa, and vanilla powder to a batter.
2. Chop the chocolate and melt it in a bain-marie (water bath). Add the coconut oil and stir until it has melted. Add the chocolate mix into the food processor bowl and mix. Press out the batter evenly in an 8-inch (20-cm) diameter springform pie pan.
3. Mix the raspberries, cashews, coconut flakes, agave syrup, and lemon juice to a smooth filling. Add in the coconut oil. Spread the filling over the pie's bottom layer and let the pie set in the freezer for about 8 hours.
4. Mix the cashews for the chocolate filling in a food processor and add the coconut oil, cocoa, and agave syrup. Mix it to a smooth cream. Spread this evenly over the raspberry filling and leave the cake in the freezer for another hour.
5. Remove the cake from the freezer about 15 minutes before serving. Top it with freeze-dried raspberries, hazelnuts, and cacao nibs.

TANGY
Cashew Balls

Full of goodness and energy, with wonderful flavor. Perfect for snacking or when you crave something really nice!

139 CALORIES/MAKES 15 BALLS

1¼ cups (3 dl) raw cashews

1¼ cups (3 dl) coconut flakes

3 tablespoons coconut flour

4 tablespoons honey

2 tablespoons fresh lemon juice

⅖ teaspoon (1½ krm) vanilla powder

2 tablespoons cold water

1¾ ounces (½ dl) dried berry powder—cranberries, raspberries, or blueberries

1. Place all the ingredients except the berry powder in a food processor and mix to a nice and smooth batter.
2. Form the batter into balls and roll to cover them in berry powder. Store in the refrigerator or freezer.

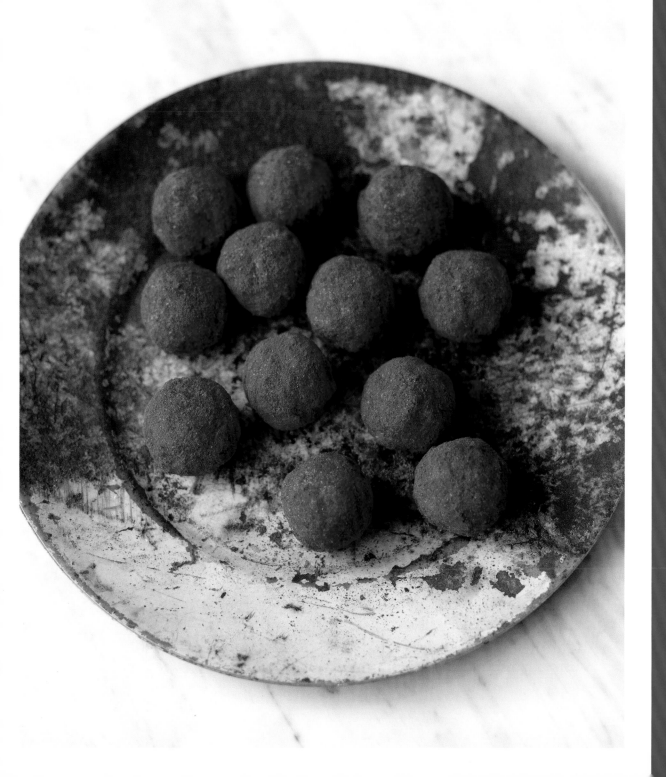

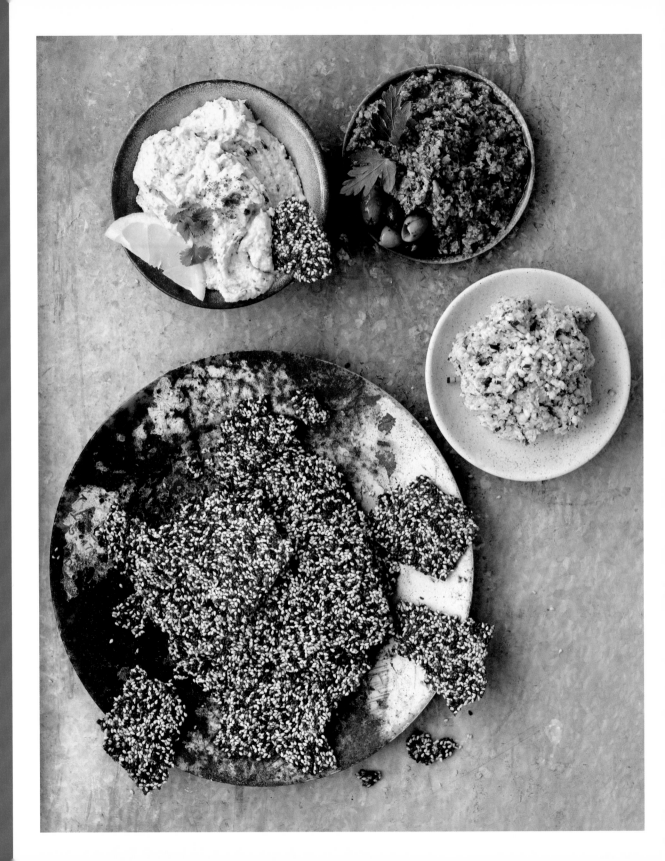

Three Tasty Dips

Why not bake a batch of Sesame Seed Crackers (p. 38) to dip in these wonderfully tasty dips?

724 CALORIES/(1 SERVING = ONE OF EACH DIP, CRACKER NOT INCLUDED) – **SERVES 4**

HUMMUS

1 can (14 ounces/400 g) chickpeas
1 clove garlic, coarsely chopped
½ bunch of cilantro
1 tablespoon sesame oil
1¾ ounces (½ dl) olive oil
Juice from ½ lemon
Salt
Black pepper

1. Drain the chickpeas in a sieve, rinse in cold water, and let drain.
2. Place the chickpeas in a food processor together with the remaining ingredients and mix to an even mixture.
3. Season with salt, pepper, and more lemon juice if desired.

CASHEW GUACAMOLE

2 avocados
3⅓ ounces (1 dl) raw cashews
1 clove garlic, coarsely chopped
½ bunch of cilantro
½ red onion, finely chopped
Juice from ½ lime
Salt
Black pepper

1. Place the avocado flesh in a food processor along with the remaining ingredients.
2. Process to a smooth mixture. Season with salt, pepper, and more lime juice if desired.

TAPENADE

3½ ounces (100 g) black and green olives, pits removed
1 small clove garlic, coarsely chopped
1¾ ounces (½ dl) parsley, chopped
1¾ fluid ounces (½ dl) olive oil
Juice from ½ lemon
Salt
Black pepper

1. Place all the ingredients in a food processor and mix to a coarse consistency.
2. Season with salt, pepper, and more lemon juice, if desired.

Chips and Brie

Crispy chips or soft and creamy goat brie?
So wonderfully yummy!

ROOT VEGETABLE CHIPS X3

147 CALORIES/SERVES 4

1 sweet potato
2 beets
3 parsnips
1 teaspoon olive oil
Persillade (parsley mixture)

1. Preheat the oven to 400°F (200°C). Brush the root vegetables thoroughly to clean, and slice them thin with a mandoline.
2. Place the vegetables on two baking sheets. Drizzle with oil and crumble the persillade over them. Mix with your hands and then spread out the slices as much as possible.
3. Roast the chips for about 20 minutes. Stir carefully once or twice during this time.
4. Remove the baking sheets from the oven and stir the chips again. Let cool.

GOAT BRIE GRATIN WITH PECANS

415 CALORIES/SERVES 4

7 ounces (200 g) goat Brie (one whole round)
3⅓ ounces (1 dl) pecans, coarsely chopped
3⅓ fluid ounces (1 dl) honey
1¾ ounces (½ dl) golden raisins

1. Preheat the oven to 437°F (225°C). Place the cheese in a small oven-safe dish.
2. Sprinkle with the nuts and drizzle with the honey. Bake in the oven about 7 to 8 minutes and then let the cheese cool a little.
3. Top with raisins and serve.

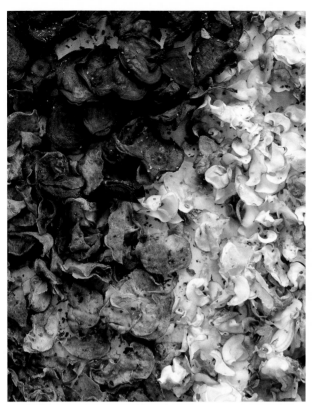

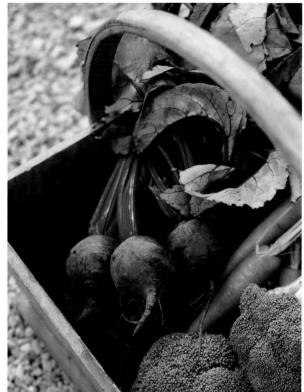

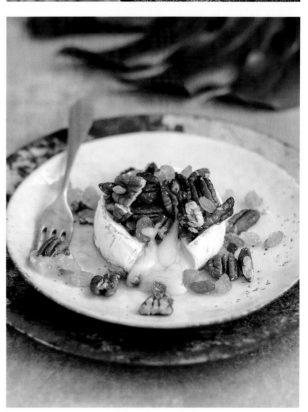

> *You can eat the goat brie as a dessert or as a snack while watching TV. It's up to you.*

Roasted
SNACKS

Is there anything nicer to snack on than slightly warm nuts and seeds? I certainly don't think so!

ROASTED SEEDS WITH PERSILLADE

135 CALORIES/SERVES 4

1¾ ounces (½ dl) slivered almonds
1¾ ounces (½ dl) pumpkin seeds
1¾ ounces (½ dl) sunflower seeds
Pinch salt flakes
⅕ teaspoon (1 krm) persillade (parsley mixture)
1 teaspoon honey

1. Heat a dry skillet and roast the slivered almonds and seeds for a few minutes while stirring.
2. Sprinkle with salt flakes and persillade, and drizzle with honey. Mix thoroughly and then pass the bowl around.

ROASTED CASHEWS WITH PECORINO CHEESE

290 CALORIES/SERVES 4

1¼ cups (3 dl) cashews
Pinch salt flakes
⅕ teaspoon (1 krm) persillade (parsley mixture)
3⅓ ounces (1 dl) finely grated pecorino cheese

1. Heat up a dry skillet and roast the cashews for a few minutes.
2. Sprinkle with salt flakes and persillade and add the grated cheese. Mix thoroughly and then pass the bowl around.

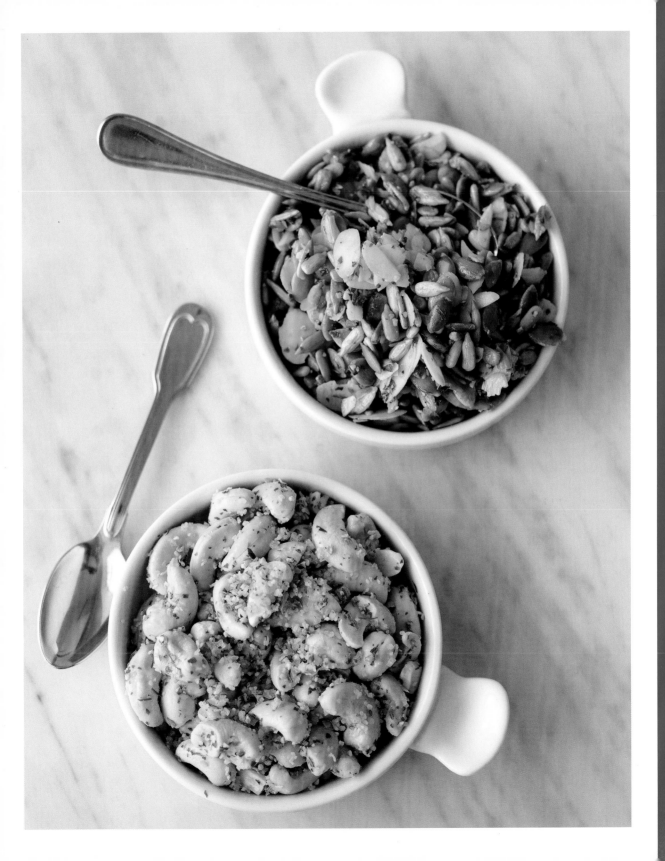

Recipe
INDEX

Subject INDEX